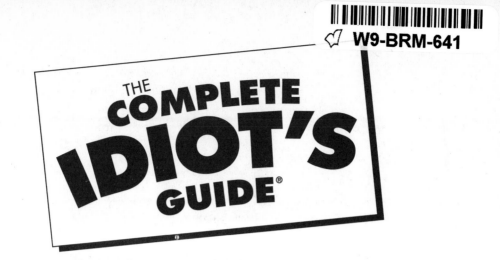

THE
COMPLETE IDIOT'S GUIDE®

Glycemic Index Cookbook

by Lucy Beale and
Joan Clark-Warner, M.S., R.D., C.D.E.

ALPHA

A member of Penguin Group (USA) Inc.

Lucy: To Patrick, Brian, Pat Jr., Christopher, Stephen, and Jessica
Joan: To my husband, Douglas

ALPHA BOOKS

Published by the Penguin Group

Penguin Group (USA) Inc., 375 Hudson Street, New York, New York 10014, USA

Penguin Group (Canada), 90 Eglinton Avenue East, Suite 700, Toronto, Ontario M4P 2Y3, Canada (a division of Pearson Penguin Canada Inc.)

Penguin Books Ltd., 80 Strand, London WC2R 0RL, England

Penguin Ireland, 25 St. Stephen's Green, Dublin 2, Ireland (a division of Penguin Books Ltd.)

Penguin Group (Australia), 250 Camberwell Road, Camberwell, Victoria 3124, Australia (a division of Pearson Australia Group Pty. Ltd.)

Penguin Books India Pvt. Ltd., 11 Community Centre, Panchsheel Park, New Delhi—110 017, India

Penguin Group (NZ), 67 Apollo Drive, Rosedale, North Shore, Auckland 1311, New Zealand (a division of Pearson New Zealand Ltd.)

Penguin Books (South Africa) (Pty.) Ltd., 24 Sturdee Avenue, Rosebank, Johannesburg 2196, South Africa

Penguin Books Ltd., Registered Offices: 80 Strand, London WC2R 0RL, England

International Standard Book Number: 978-1-59257-861-0
Library of Congress Catalog Card Number: 2008935071

11   10   09   8   7   6   5   4   3   2   1

Interpretation of the printing code: The rightmost number of the first series of numbers is the year of the book's printing; the rightmost number of the second series of numbers is the number of the book's printing. For example, a printing code of 09-1 shows that the first printing occurred in 2009.

Printed in the United States of America

Note: This publication contains the opinions and ideas of its authors. It is intended to provide helpful and informative material on the subject matter covered. It is sold with the understanding that the authors and publisher are not engaged in rendering professional services in the book. If the reader requires personal assistance or advice, a competent professional should be consulted.

Most Alpha books are available at special quantity discounts for bulk purchases for sales promotions, premiums, fund-raising, or educational use. Special books, or book excerpts, can also be created to fit specific needs.

For details, write: Special Markets, Alpha Books, 375 Hudson Street, New York, NY 10014.

Publisher: *Marie Butler-Knight*
Editorial Director: *Mike Sanders*
Senior Managing Editor: *Billy Fields*
Acquisitions Editor: *Tom Stevens*
Development Editor: *Nancy D. Lewis*
Senior Production Editor: *Janette Lynn*
Copy Editor: *Jan Zoya*

Cover Designer: *Rebecca Harmon*
Book Designer: *Trina Wurst*
Indexer: *Angie Bess*
Layout: *Ayanna Lacey*
Proofreader: *John Etchison*

Contents at a Glance

Contents

13 Pork, Lamb, and Veal Main Dishes   131

14 Poultry Main Dishes   147

Introduction

Cooking based on the glycemic index is inspiring. You'll be doing something valuable for yourself, your family, and friends with each meal you prepare. Often, you'll find the meals from this cookbook taste better because you'll be using many fresh farm-sourced ingredients and interesting spices, herbs, and condiments.

In addition, you'll find you won't be spending more time in the kitchen, but that your cooking will be more effective at supporting your health and slimming your waistline.

We designed this cookbook to fit into a busy lifestyle that includes work and evening/weekend activities. You'll find chapters with quick breakfast recipes and one with take-along snacks. Our recipes will accommodate anyone—from a person who sits down for three square meals a day to one who lives with an irregular schedule and time demands.

If you've chosen this cookbook for yourself or to prepare meals for a family member, know that you can confidently feed the whole family with the recipes in this book. In fact, these recipes don't taste like diet food at all. They're that delicious!

If you have a sweet tooth and love desserts, you'll find satisfaction in the three chapters of sweet endings that are low to medium glycemic. Every chocolate devotee will treasure the dessert chapter devoted entirely to chocolate.

In writing this cookbook, we enjoyed creating delectable recipes that can improve health, support weight loss, and taste good. We've both eaten low glycemic for over 10 years and can tell you from our hearts that it's been worth it every bite of the way.

How This Book Is Organized

This book is divided into six parts:

Part 1, "Cooking the Glycemic Index Way" explains the health and weight-loss benefits of eating and cooking based on the glycemic index. You'll learn how to identify high, medium, and low glycemic value foods and understand glycemic load while using the Plate Method of creating balanced meals. Stock your pantry with farm-sourced low-glycemic foods.

Part 2, "Good Starts and Snacks," offers you recipes for quick breakfasts and leisurely breakfasts. You'll enjoy delicious breads and find solutions for low-glycemic take-along snacks.

Part 3, "On the Light Side," answers the question of what to eat for lunches, appetizers, and snacks. Sauces and condiments give you many ways to jazz up your meals with savory or sweet enhancements. Enjoy soups that can serve as main dishes or accompaniments.

Part 4, "Main Dishes," contains recipes for salads, beef, pork, lamb, veal, poultry, and seafood that range from simple to elegant. We've added a chapter on low-glycemic vegetarian main dishes, too.

Part 5, "On the Side," gives you recipes for delicious side dishes—salads, vegetables, fruit, potatoes, and grains.

Part 6, "Sweet Endings," offers you recipes to satisfy your sweet tooth with fruit desserts, chocolate desserts, cakes, pies, cookies, and puddings.

Extras

We know you're embarking on a new way of thinking about foods and cooking. To boost your confidence and knowledge, this book contains special messages that offer tips, tricks, and tidbits to help you along the way. Look for these elements that will enhance your cooking:

Tasty Tidbits

Use these tips and hints to create delicious eating.

def•i•ni•tion

With these definitions you'll be glycemic-savvy in the kitchen and in eating.

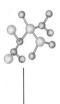

Glycemic Notes

Use these meal preparation and nutrition suggestions so that your expertise never falters.

Home-Cooked Goodness

Gain information about cooking techniques and the application of the glycemic index to your meals.

Acknowledgments

Lucy and Joan give special thanks to their families, clients, and friends, who have inspired them to create recipes that make glycemic eating delectable, tasty, and easy.

Lucy Beale thanks her husband, Patrick, for his helpful support and meal preparation while she was occupied and preoccupied with writing. She also thanks her stepson, Pat Jr., for grammar and editing assistance. Lucy thanks her co-author, Joan, for her careful nutritional calculations and insightful recipe recommendations.

Joan Clark-Warner thanks her husband, Douglas, for his patience and kindness while she edited and wrote nutrition information, and calculated nutrient analysis for the recipes. She also thanks her children, Jenny, Ryan, and Tricia, for their encouragement. And she thanks the author, Lucy, for her expertise, enthusiasm, and creativity.

Lucy and Joan both thank Marilyn Allen of the Allen O'Shea Literary Agency and Tom Stephens, editor at Alpha Books, for guiding this book from inception through publication. Special thanks to Jennie Brand-Miller for permission to excerpt the glycemic index from her book *What Makes My Blood Glucose Go Up ... and Down?* written with Kaye Foster-Powell and Rick Mendosa. And to Rick Mendosa for creating www.mendosa.com, which offers valuable and practical information on the glycemic index.

Special Thanks to the Technical Reviewer

The Complete Idiot's Guide Glycemic Index Cookbook was reviewed by an expert who double-checked the accuracy of what you'll learn here, to help us ensure that this book gives you everything you need to know about cooking according to the glycemic index. Special thanks are extended to Lisa Vislocky.

Trademarks

Part 1

Cooking Based on the Glycemic Index

Get set for fun cooking and great eating with the glycemic index as your inspiration. In addition to learning about the many health and weight-loss benefits, you'll learn an accessible way to eat balanced meals using the Plate Method.

Use farm-sourced foods when possible and avoid highly processed factory-sourced foods to get the most nutritional and gustatory pleasure from each bite.

Cooking the Glycemic Index Way

In This Chapter

- ◆ Low-glycemic eating for taste and health
- ◆ Menu planning for meals and snacks
- ◆ The plate method of dishing

As you read this cookbook, you'll find that cooking based on the glycemic index comes easily to you. The cooking techniques are the same ones you use now. What's different are the proportions of ingredients and the use of more natural grains and starches.

You won't need to make excuses or apologies to company, friends, and family about your low-glycemic meals—the food will be just as savory, delicious, and satisfying as the meals you've made before. And expect rave reviews—glycemic index cooks dish up some of the best and most healthful ingredients in wonderful ways.

Palate-Pleasing Meals

Glycemic index eating is a treat, and you'll soon discover that low-glycemic eating isn't a burdensome challenge. You'll receive benefits that help you lose weight, manage your blood sugar levels, and reduce insulin resistance and metabolic syndrome. You'll also be eating meals that are enjoyable and satisfying to your palate as well as to your waistline.

We've designed these recipes to fit into your lifestyle and your existing eating habits. You'll find special chapters on quick breakfasts, snacks, appetizers, and lunches, and entire chapters devoted to chocolate and desserts.

Health-Promoting Foods

For over 20 years, the glycemic index has been helping people lose weight, reduce metabolic syndrome, and manage blood sugar levels. Here are some of those potential health benefits:

- Weight loss and weight management

- Improved skin tone with fewer wrinkles and sagging

- Smaller waist and flatter tummy

- Healthy management of type 2 diabetes in combination with exercise and possibly without medication

- Prevention of diabetes and/or metabolic syndrome

- Lower stress levels

Eating low glycemic can do all of the above because it helps keep your blood sugar levels and insulin levels in the healthy range.

Low vs. High-Glycemic Carbohydrates

It's very simple: eating mostly *high-glycemic carbohydrates* is not beneficial to your health, while eating mostly low-glycemic carbohydrates is beneficial. High-glycemic carbohydrates cause a quick spike in the fat-storing hormone insulin, and a quick rise in blood sugar levels. Examples of high-glycemic carbohydrates are white breads, bagels, rice crackers, frozen-yogurt desserts, popcorn, baked white potatoes, and often the treat foods of candy, cakes, and cookies. Some baked goods can be medium glycemic if they contain enough fat to slow digestion of high-glycemic components such as flour.

Low-glycemic carbohydrates include fruits, vegetables, and legumes. Coarsely ground whole grains, natural stone-ground bread, yams, some varieties of rice, and peanuts are also low glycemic. Meat, seafood, and fat eaten in a balanced diet are effectively zero glycemic and have little to no effect on your insulin levels.

def•i•ni•tion

High-glycemic carbohydrates are often made from white flours, or even some finely milled whole wheat flours. Other high-glycemic carbohydrates include white potatoes, puffed rice, and popcorn. They may also include large amounts of sugar or high-fructose corn syrup.

Medium-glycemic foods fall in between. You can eat some—but not lots—of these foods, which include many whole grains, moderately processed products containing cornmeal, whole wheat, some varieties of rice, and processed oats. Sweet corn, beets, and canned fruits packed in sugar are medium glycemic.

This may sound as if eating low glycemic is uninteresting and borders on self-deprivation and culinary boredom. It isn't, as the recipes give you scrumptious, anything-but-boring meals. You'll find ways to eat chocolate, desserts, and snacks in a balanced way so you receive the many benefits of eating low glycemic. For balanced eating, include some high- and medium-glycemic foods with a meal that includes meats, eggs, or fish, and fruits and vegetables.

To quickly help determine if a food is high glycemic, use these two rules-of-the-waistline: "white and fluffy makes you puffy," and "if it's gooey and sticky, be real picky." Mostly avoid those sorts of foods.

Insulin, Health, and Inflammation

When you eat a normal-size serving of a high-glycemic carbohydrate by itself without a balanced meal, the levels of your fat-storing hormone, insulin, rise along with your blood sugar levels. This sets off a series of metabolic processes that can possibly result in the following:

 ◆ Loss of the ability of your body's cells to uptake glucose—also known as insulin resistance—which could lead to metabolic syndrome and type 2 diabetes

 ◆ Weight gain, especially around your waistline

◆ Generalized inflammation that can cause constriction of artery walls, leading to heart disease

◆ Increase in the stress hormone cortisol, thus increasing your stress levels

◆ Acceleration of the signs of aging: wrinkles; loss of muscle tone on face; loss of muscle tone in other parts of the body including legs, torso, arms

◆ Inflammation that promotes or worsens autoimmune disorders

◆ Anxiety, depression, or mood swings

To learn about more research on the glycemic index and its health benefits, go to www.glycemicindex.com.

If you have any of these situations, eating a mostly low-glycemic diet can help your body to improve or prevent the condition. If you suspect that you have any of these conditions, consult with your health practitioner.

The Glycemic Index Scale

Using the glycemic index can take numerous arithmetic calculations to figure out the glycemic index of just one meal. On the one hand, this is good, because the glycemic index is thoroughly based on science. But it's also bad, because you have better things to do with your time and mental energy than make the calculations, and it can make a low-glycemic food plan seem like too great a challenge.

In these recipes, we've made things simple. We give you four rankings:

High-glycemic recipes are over 70 on the glycemic index scale.

Medium-glycemic are between 55 to 69.

Low-glycemic are between 10-54.

Very low-glycemic are below 10.

We've also included other important nutritional information with each recipe, including grams of fat, fiber, carbs, and protein and amount of calories.

Elements of a Balanced Meal

Forget your grade school food pyramid—we know more about food today and how it fuels or harms your body. Today's balanced meal requires plenty of vegetables and fruit, protein, and good fats. At each meal—breakfast, lunch, and dinner—plan on eating the following:

- 1 (3- to 4-ounce) serving of a *complete protein:* meat, poultry, seafood, eggs, or cheese

def•i•ni•tion

Complete protein, also known as high-quality protein, contains adequate amounts of all nine essential amino acids. The following foods contain complete protein: beef, poultry, seafood, other meats, eggs, and cheese. Milk contains complete protein but in lower concentration. Vegetable protein, such as soy or legumes, does not have as high a biological value as animal protein and is not as easy to digest and assimilate.

- 2 to 3 servings of vegetables or fruit (a serving is ½ cup cooked or 1 cup raw)
- 1 to 2 tablespoons of good fats, such as olive oil or the fat contained in foods such as avocados, meats, nuts, and seeds
- 1 serving low-glycemic starches or grains

You can't go wrong nutritionally eating green vegetables, but you can go wrong overeating any of the food basics: carbohydrates, fats, or proteins.

Glycemic Load

To help you balance your meals well, we've added glycemic load calculations to each recipe. The glycemic load factors how much and what type of carbohydrate you eat so that you can best manage your weight and health.

A normal healthy person's daily glycemic load can be between 138 and 163. If you are very physically active, you can handle a higher glycemic load. If you want to lose weight, or want to manage blood sugar levels, you need to eat below 138 daily.

To find the glycemic load that works best for you, you'll need to experiment, starting with a low value of about 100, and increasing it until you are meeting your weight loss or health goals.

The Plate Method of Balanced Eating

Here's what to dish up on your plate:

- ♦ About ¹/₂ your plate should contain nonstarchy vegetables such as salads, tomatoes, green beans

- ♦ About ¹/₄ is a lean protein—meats, poultry, eggs, cheese, seafood

- ♦ ¹/₈ is for good fats: olive oil, butter, or the fats in salad dressing and sauces

- ♦ ¹/₄ is for fruit, low-glycemic starches, or dairy

We doubt your plate will always work out this way, because you'll be eating combined foods such as stews, soups, sandwiches, and salads.

Home-Cooked Goodness

When using the plate method, if you want dessert, save room on your plate and in your stomach. Don't fill your plate completely with your meal. Dessert is usually included in the one fourth that contains dairy, fruit, or starches.

Eating low-glycemic can easily become a way of life for you and your family. You don't need to give up much in terms of food choices, and you'll be replacing less-nutritious high-glycemic carbohydrates with comparable, more healthful low-glycemic food selections.

In time you'll find, as we did, that you'll never return to your old ways of having coffee and pastry for breakfast, a cookie with diet soda for lunch, then eating everything in the pantry for dinner and beyond until bed. You'll be eating well and enjoying the results.

The Least You Need to Know

- ♦ Low-glycemic cooking is healthful and a delight to your palate.

- ♦ Eating low glycemic is shown to reduce insulin resistance and inflammation.

- ♦ Weight loss and weight management are easy when eating based on the glycemic index and glycemic load.

- ♦ Avoid eating "white and fluffy foods" and limit "gooey and sticky foods" as they are usually high glycemic.

Stocking Your Glycemic Index Kitchen

In This Chapter

◆ Staples for your pantry and refrigerator

◆ Shopping for ingredients

◆ Kitchen tools and techniques

Right now, this very minute, you can prepare a delicious low- to medium-glycemic meal with ingredients you already have in your kitchen. (We're assuming that you prepare meals on a regular basis.) All you need are some kind of complete protein and fresh, frozen, or canned vegetables.

Ah, but man or woman does not thrive on plain and boring food alone. You've been there, done that. Let's change the paradigm so you can prepare wonderful meals by stocking your pantry with staples that spice up both your meals and life.

Wise Ingredient Selections

In writing this cookbook and creating the recipes, we focused on selecting ingredients that provide you with the utmost in healthy nutrition from the most delicious and delectable foods including low-glycemic carbohydrates.

Most ingredients in the recipes are farm-sourced. This means that they are unprocessed or minimally processed. They're widely available, and with just a few exceptions can be purchased at your local grocery store or health food store. If any of the ingredients aren't available locally, you can purchase them on the Internet. We give you the specifics in Appendix A.

To explain our choices of ingredients, refer to the Glycemic Index Food Source Chart. Here are the main features of the chart:

◆ On the vertical axis is the glycemic index, ranging from low glycemic, 0 to 55, to medium glycemic, 56 to 69, on up to high glycemic, 70 and above.

◆ On the horizontal axis is a range of food categories: farm-sourced, processed with nutritional value, processed with low or no nutritional value, and factory-sourced with additives/mystery ingredients. The foods to the left are the most wholesome and natural; the foods to the right are the most highly processed and contain the most artificial ingredients.

◆ Each area of the graph contains a letter: A, B, C, A2, B2, C2, D, or F1, F2, and F3.

◆ The recipes use mainly A, B, and A2 foods, with a couple others used occasionally for sweetness or baking. We don't use F-foods in our recipes.

A-sector foods are the healthiest for you to eat and are the foods used universally in our recipes. They include low-glycemic farm-sourced foods, such as vegetables, fruits, meat, eggs, fish, poultry, most honey, legumes, yams, sweet potatoes, thick-cut oatmeal, nuts, and seeds. Also included are minimally processed foods such as herbs, spices, pickles, horseradish, sun-dried tomatoes, most dried fruit, and other condiments. Dairy products—milk, cheese, yogurt, and sour cream that don't contain additives and preservatives are A-sector foods, as are coffee and tea.

B-sector foods are healthful but medium glycemic. They include beets, fresh corn, basmati rice, cantaloupe, pineapple, wild rice, and stone-ground bread.

C-sector foods are high glycemic, but still farm-sourced. Our recipes seldom call for C-sector foods. They aren't great for low-glycemic eating, except in small amounts eaten with foods that are low glycemic. C-sector foods include white potatoes, millet, all-natural popcorn, parsnips, and rutabagas. Isn't it interesting that not many farm-sourced foods are high glycemic?

High Glycemic	White potatoes Millet Popcorn Tapioca	Grape nuts Whole wheat blended bread, finely milled	White bread Pretzels Rice cakes Bagel	Some protein bars Frozen soy desserts Gatorade Sodas Donuts Most boxed breakfast cereal French fries Crackers High-fructose corn syrup
70	**C**	**C2**	**D**	**F3**
Medium Glycemic 69	Corn meal Raisins Figs Pineapple Wild rice	Some 100% grain breakfast cereals	Table sugar Instant oatmeal Brown sugar	Some candy Juice cocktail Some protein bars Potato chips
56	**B**	**B2**	**D**	**F2**
Low Glycemic 55	Oat Bran Basmati rice New potatoes Dates Legumes Sweet potato Slow-cook oatmeal Milk, barley Most fruit Most vegetables Meat, seafood, nuts, eggs, cheese	Coarsely ground whole wheat bread Milk chocolate Ice cream Dark chocolate 100% Juice	Soy protein isolate	Soy milk Nonfat sugar-free fruit yogurts Trans fats Artificial sweeteners Diet Sodas
0	**A**	**A2**	**D**	**F1**
	Farm-Sourced Foods	**Processed with Nutritional Value**	**Processed with Low-Nutritional Value**	**Factory-Source Foods-additives, "mystery" ingredients**

Glycemic Index Food Source Chart.

A2-sector foods are minimally processed low-glycemic foods with great nutritional value. They include 100 percent juice, coarsely ground whole-wheat and stone-ground breads, dark and milk chocolate, and pure, all-natural ice cream.

B2-sector foods are naturally processed medium-glycemic food. In this category are some 100 percent whole-grain breakfast cereals.

C2-sector foods are natural, processed, and high glycemic. These include Grape Nuts and fluffy whole-wheat bread made with finely milled grain.

D-sector foods are processed foods with low to no nutritional value. They definitely aren't nutrient dense so you may not want to waste room in your stomach on D-sector foods when you could eat more nourishing fare. They aren't helpful for weight loss and health because they don't deliver value. They're far removed from being farm-sourced.

Foods in the F-sector flunk. They're diet and health destroyers and need to be eaten with caution, if at all. Preferably, you'd avoid them.

F1 foods flunk. Yes, they're low glycemic, but that's all they have going for them. Avoid these. They're full of mystery ingredients or artificial sweeteners. They include diet sodas, zero-calorie drink mixes, artificially sweetened diet foods such as yogurt and cookies, soy milk, most beef jerky (unless it's totally natural), and corn dogs.

F2 foods also flunk. They're medium-glycemic and full of mystery ingredients. These include frozen dinners, some candy, some protein bars, potato chips, juice cocktails, donuts, potato chips, and corn chips.

F3 foods really flunk. They give you a double whammy of bad: high-glycemic foods filled with mystery ingredients. No amount of nutritionally healthy eating can make up for eating too many F3 foods. These include frozen soy desserts, sugary boxed cereals, sodas, colas, electrolyte-replenishment drinks like Gatorade, high-caffeine sodas, popsicles, candy like jelly beans, many protein bars and power bars, french fries, and many other "treat" foods.

By using mostly farm-sourced low-glycemic foods as ingredients in our recipes, you know that you're eating high-quality food with high levels of nutrition and value.

The Cupboard's Not Bare or Boring

Keeping your pantry stocked with glycemic-savvy foods will let you make a meal quickly without resorting to high-glycemic fast food or salsa and chips for dinner. You don't need to purchase all of these ingredients today, but over time you can stock your pantry with these types of foods, based on your personal preferences:

◆ Canned tuna, sardines, clams, and salmon

◆ Whole-wheat pasta

◆ Jars of tomato-based spaghetti sauce, preferably the brand with the fewest *mystery ingredients*

◆ Olive oil

def•i•ni•tion

Mystery ingredients are the ingredients on the label that you can't pronounce, don't really know what they are, aren't food-based products, are artificial sweeteners, or are preservatives and colorings. As much as possible, avoid purchasing or eating products with mystery ingredients. Researchers simply don't know their long-term health implications.

- A selection of herbal teas that you enjoy

- An assortment of spices and herbs, including tarragon, cayenne powder, oregano, rosemary, garlic salt, fennel seed, ginger, red pepper flakes, parsley, cinnamon, chili powder, basil, and others you enjoy. Be sure to stock salt and black peppercorns.

Tasty Tidbits _____

Hot spices such as chiles, chili powder, and cayenne help you lose weight by increasing your metabolism. They lower your cravings for fatty foods and sweets and increase your sense of well-being by releasing endorphins. You'll find plenty of recipes here that include chiles and hot spices. You can add less or more than called for, based on your taste preference.

- Basmati rice, wild rice, brown rice

- Dried fruit, such as cranberries, raisins, dates, figs

- A selection of nuts and seeds—pecans, peanuts, walnuts, almonds, filberts, sunflower seeds, sesame seeds, pumpkin seeds, pinions, pistachios, and others you enjoy.

- Peanut butter and perhaps almond or cashew butter (for quick, high-energy balanced snacks, serve with fruit)

- Canned vegetables and condiments: black olives, marinated artichoke hearts, tomato and chili sauce, whole tomatoes, diced green chiles, vinegars, and olive oil

Add to your pantry some of your favorite canned goods, such as artichoke hearts; beets; whole tomatoes; and beans such as garbanzo, kidney, black, and pinto beans.

Foods NOT to keep in your house are such high-glycemic convenience foods as Spaghetti-Os, rice crackers, popcorn, white bread, white crackers, and sodas—diet or regular.

Acidic and Sour Foods

We've added recipes that include many acidic and sour foods, because they are super-important for your weight loss and health success. Simply by eating a sour or acidic food with each meal, you can lower the total glycemic effect of the meal by as much as one third and better support your weight-loss or health efforts.

Glycemic Notes _____

Some commercial breads are low glycemic. Purchase stone-ground bread—the kind that's heavy and not white or fluffy. Beware of packaged breads that claim to be whole-wheat or stone-ground. If they're light and fluffy, use caution. Read the ingredients list and you'll probably find white flour, wheat flour, or a finely milled flour that boosts the glycemic index value of the bread. Avoid breads with caramel coloring that makes the bread look healthier than it is. The only exception is sourdough bread. Its acidic/sour taste makes it low glycemic. The more sour, the better.

Sour foods slow the absorption of sugars in your stomach, thus helping you prevent a quick rise in blood sugar and the accompanying rise in the fat-storing hormone insulin.

Some people love sour foods; for others they're an acquired taste. Here's a list of sour foods and condiments you can enjoy:

◆ Capers

◆ Chutney

◆ Coffee and black tea

◆ Dill pickles

◆ Grapefruit

◆ Green olives

◆ Hershey's baking chocolate and cocoa that's NOT Dutch processed. This is unsweetened and very bitter.

◆ Horseradish

◆ Lemon and lime juice (purchase at health food stores in bottles that don't contain preservatives or additives, but are simply pure juice)

◆ Sauerkraut

◆ Marinated vegetables, such as artichokes, carrots, broccoli, Brussels sprouts

◆ Pickled beets, legumes, onions, or garlic

◆ Pickled eggs

◆ Pickled herring

- Salsas made with vinegar

- Sauerbraten

- Sourdough bread (the tangier the better)

- Tangy condiments and relishes, such as olive spread, sun-dried tomato spreads, tomato-onion relish, and others

- Vinaigrette salad dressings

- Vinegar

If you pass up sour foods at a meal, you can easily add a couple squeezes of lemon to a glass of water and drink with or after your meal.

Sweeteners

Sweeteners are controversial. Some people fear them; others avoid them altogether.

The recipes in our cookbook call for natural sweeteners, because they're the best for baking and cooking, and because we've figured out how to make a little go a long way. Natural sweeteners contain calories and not much nutritional value, but we prefer them to artificial ones. We'll show you how to cook with them to keep the calorie count low and the glycemic effect as low as possible. Here are the sweeteners to purchase:

- White table sugar is the standard by which all other sweeteners are measured for taste, browning, and baking. Table sugar is medium glycemic.

- Fructose. This fruit sugar comes in granulated form. It's low glycemic.

Glycemic Notes _____

Don't confuse granulated fructose for baking with high-fructose corn syrup. High-fructose corn syrup is a suspect in chronic health conditions, such as heart disease, metabolic syndrome, and diabetes. It's present in many soft drinks, electrolyte beverages, packaged candies, baked goods, and snack foods.

- Xylitol is a sugar alcohol that blends well with table sugar, is low glycemic, and offers some excellent health benefits.

Home-Cooked Goodness

Xylitol is used in chewing gum and may reduce bacteria in the mouth and gums. It's low glycemic and contains only 40 percent of the calories of table sugar.

◆ Stevia is a very low-glycemic herb from South America that's very sweet and can be purchased in the health food section of grocery stores or in health food stores.

◆ Pure honey is usually low glycemic and very sweet.

◆ Molasses is the dark, rich-tasting syrup of the sugarcane plant.

With these six sweeteners used sparingly, you can satisfy your sweet tooth in a glycemic-savvy way.

The Least You Need to Know

◆ Stock your kitchen with low-glycemic foods and healthful ingredients for ease of meal preparation and for quick meals.

◆ Keep plenty of acidic/sour foods and condiments on hand and serve with meals to lower the glycemic effect of your food.

◆ Shorten meal preparation time by using helpful kitchen equipment.

Part 2

Good Starts and Snacks

Breakfast is a most important meal, so we show you how to catch a superb low-glycemic breakfast on the run. When you have more time, create a leisurely breakfast from our scrumptious recipes. And don't worry if you need to eat low-fat, we've provided low-fat variations for some of the recipes.

Breads aren't off limits for low-glycemic eating. Bake up these glorious loaves and muffins and you'll appreciate their earthy goodness.

We give you answers for take-along snacks. You'll gain quick energy that can hold you for hours as you eat snacks that don't require refrigeration or special attention.

Quick Breakfasts

In This Chapter

- ◆ Breakfast is your powerful assist
- ◆ A little planning and a lot of value
- ◆ Appetizing and fast

Breakfast is so essential to your health and well-being that we've devoted two chapters to breakfast recipes: quick breakfasts and leisurely breakfasts.

To qualify as a quick breakfast, the preparation and cook time needed to be less than 15 minutes combined, and preferably lower than that. We figure you should be able to whip up a good breakfast in the time it takes to brew a pot of coffee.

You'll find plenty of favorites and some that you can carry with you to the office or gym. New scientific research targets our need for breakfast, even whole eggs.

Ham and Cheese Omelet

Yields one 2-egg omelet
Prep time: 3 minutes
Cook time: 4 minutes
Serving size: 2 eggs and ¼ cup ham
Each serving:
Glycemic index: very low
Glycemic load: 0
Calories: 284
Protein: 25 grams
Carbohydrates: 0 grams
Fiber: 0 grams
Fat: 23 grams
Saturated fat: 8.8 grams

A classic breakfast omelet with the delicious flavors of ham and Parmesan cheese.

2 eggs

¼ cup diced 5 percent lean ham

2 TB. chopped onion

¼ tsp. basil

⅛ tsp. freshly ground black pepper

2 TB. Parmesan cheese

1 TB. olive oil

1. Whisk eggs in a medium-size bowl. Stir in diced ham and onion. Add basil, pepper, and parmesan cheese.

2. Heat olive oil in a small skillet. Pour in egg mixture and cook until one side is lightly browned. Flip and cook the other side until golden brown.

Eggs with Tarragon Sauce

Yields 2 eggs plus 1 cup sauce
Prep time: 5 minutes
Cook time: 10 minutes
Serving size: 1 egg plus 1 TB. sauce
Each serving:
Glycemic index: very low
Glycemic load: 0
Calories: 212
Protein: 7 grams
Carbohydrates: 0 grams
Fiber: 0 grams
Fat: 20.4 grams
Saturated fat: 5.5 grams

A delightfully tangy and lightly peppery rich sauce for morning eggs.

2 TB. mayonnaise

2 tsp. butter, melted

½ tsp. Dijon mustard

½ tsp. dried tarragon

1 tsp. lemon juice

⅛ tsp. salt

⅛ tsp. freshly ground black pepper

2 eggs

1. Whisk together mayonnaise, butter, mustard, tarragon, lemon juice, salt, and pepper.

2. Cook eggs to your preference: poached, fried, scramble, etc.

3. Spoon 1 tablespoon sauce on each egg and serve.

4. Store any leftover sauce in a jar with a tight-fitting lid and refrigerate.

Yogurt-Layered Breakfast Salad

Creamy, sweet, and crunchy goodness for a quick breakfast treat.

½ cup 2 percent cottage cheese

¼ cup granola

¼ cup plain low-fat yogurt

½ cup mixed fresh berries

2 TB. coarsely chopped walnuts

2 TB. raisins

1 TB. honey

Yields 1½ cups salad
Prep time: 5 minutes
Cook time: none
Serving size: 1½ cups salad
Each serving:
Glycemic index: low
Glycemic load: 30
Calories: 423
Protein: 24 grams
Carbohydrates: 61 grams
Fiber: 4 grams
Fat: 9.2 grams
Saturated fat: 2 grams

1. In an individual serving bowl, layer ingredients: put half of the cottage cheese on bottom, top with half the granola, then half the yogurt, half the berries, half the walnuts, half the raisins, and repeat.

2. Drizzle honey on top of all and serve.

Variation: Substitute any fruit for the berries, any nut for the walnuts, and any dried fruit for the raisins.

The Easiest Quick Breakfast We Know

Savor the taste of a fresh egg with salt and pepper eaten with ripe fresh fruit.

1 tsp. olive oil

1 egg (or 2, if you're hungry)

1 medium-size apple, pear, or orange

Yields 1 egg and fruit
Prep time: 2 minutes
Cook time: 3 minutes
Serving size: full recipe
Each serving:
Glycemic index: low
Glycemic load: 11
Calories: 242
Protein: 8 grams (two eggs = 15 g)
Carbohydrates: 30 grams
Fiber: 3 grams
Fat: 10 grams
Saturated fat: 2.2 grams

1. Heat olive oil over low-medium heat in a small cast-iron skillet. Break egg into the pan and cook until egg whites turn opaque. Break yolk with fork and turn egg. Cook 3 seconds.

2. Slice fruit into wedges. Put egg and fruit on a plate.

Home-Cooked Goodness

We gave you directions for a fried egg, but you can make whatever type of egg you prefer: over-medium, over-easy, poached, sunny-side up. Other fruit options include grapes, any type of berry, peaches, plums, and nectarines.

Sweet Raspberry Crepe

Yields 6 egg pancakes
Prep time: 5 minutes
Cook time: 8 minutes
Serving size: 1½ eggs and ¼ cup berries
Each serving:
Glycemic index: low
Glycemic load: 5
Calories: 222
Protein: 11 grams
Carbohydrates: 12 grams
Fiber: 1 gram
Fat: 14.5 grams
Saturated fat: 4.77 grams

The slightly sweet, thick crepe holds a slightly tangy raspberry sauce.

1 cup defrosted frozen raspberries	**½ tsp. salt**
3 tsp. sugar	**¼ cup water**
6 eggs	**¼ cup low-fat milk**
2 TB. cornstarch	**1 TB. butter**
	1 TB. olive oil

1. In a small bowl, mix berries with 1 teaspoon sugar and set aside.

2. In a mixing bowl, beat eggs with 2 teaspoons sugar, cornstarch, salt, water, and milk.

3. Heat butter and olive oil in a skillet over medium heat. Pour batter into the pan and cook as an omelet, browning on both sides.

4. Divide pancake into 6 plates. Top each serving with ¼ cup berries.

Eggs with Spinach and Cheese

Yields 8 eggs plus spinach and cheese
Prep time: 5 minutes
Cook time: 6 minutes
Serving size: 2 eggs each
Each serving:
Glycemic index: very low
Glycemic load: 0
Calories: 247
Protein: 14 grams
Carbohydrates: <1 gram
Fiber: <1 gram
Fat: 21 grams
Saturated fat: 6.95 grams

Spinach delivers vegetable flavor combined with the mild cheese taste of Monterey Jack.

8 large eggs	**2 oz. Monterey Jack cheese, shredded**
2 TB. olive oil	**Dash salt and freshly ground black pepper**
1 cup baby spinach leaves, coarsely chopped	

1. In a bowl, gently beat eggs until blended.

2. Heat olive oil in a large skillet over medium heat. Add beaten eggs and cook, stirring several times, until eggs begin to solidify, 1½–2 minutes. Add spinach and cheese, stir once or twice, and continue to cook until mixture is softly firm. Sprinkle with salt and pepper to taste. Serve.

Quick Steel-Cut Oatmeal

Cinnamon, raisins, and cottage cheese provide fragrant flavor the low-glycemic steel-cut oats.

¼ cup steel-cut oats, not long-cooking or instant oatmeal

¾ cup water

½ tsp. cinnamon

1 TB. raisins

½ cup low-fat cottage cheese

Yields 1½ cups cereal
Prep time: 2 minutes
Cook time: 8 minutes
Serving size: 1½ cups
Each serving:
Glycemic index: low
Glycemic load: 15
Calories: 248
Protein: 20 grams
Carbohydrates: 37 grams
Fiber: 4 grams
Fat: 2.2 grams
Saturated fat: 1.4 grams

1. Add steel-cut oats to water in a deep, large microwavable bowl. The oats will bubble up, so using a deep bowl is important.

2. Microwave on high for 5 minutes. Stir. Return to the microwave and cook on high for 3 minutes.

3. Remove from the microwave and stir in cinnamon, raisins, and cottage cheese, then serve.

On-the-Run Breakfast

Hard-boiled eggs were designed for busy people. Eat with ripe fruit and you have a meal.

1 egg, hard-boiled

1 medium fruit, such as apple, pear, bunch of grapes, nectarine

Yields 1 egg and 1 piece fruit
Prep time: 1 minute
Cook time: none
Serving size: 1 egg and 1 piece fruit
Each serving:
Glycemic index: low
Glycemic load: 11
Calories: 197
Protein: 8 grams
Carbohydrates: 30 grams
Fiber: 3 grams
Fat: 5 grams
Saturated fat: 1.6 grams

1. Hard-boil eggs up to a week ahead. To hard-boil: Place up to a dozen eggs in a saucepan. Cover with water. Bring to a boil. Cover eggs with a saucepan lid, and turn off heat. Let stand in the very hot water for 6 minutes or longer. Remove from the stove. Run cold water over eggs until they're cooled enough to touch. Refrigerate until ready to eat.

2. To fix breakfast: peel egg, and place in brown bag with fruit and napkin.

Office Eggs

Yields 2 eggs
Prep time: 2 minutes
Cook time: 2 minutes
Serving size: 2 eggs
Each serving:
Glycemic index: low
Glycemic load: 11
Calories: 270
Protein: 15 grams
Carbohydrates: 30 grams
Fiber: 3 grams
Fat: 10 grams
Saturated fat: 3 grams

Microwaving scrambled eggs dressed up with your favorite spices, herbs, or additions is a winner at your morning break.

2 eggs

Dash salt and black pepper

1 piece fruit, such as apple, pear, peach

1. Before you go to work, break eggs into a microwavable container with a tight-fitting lid. Season with your favorite herbs or spices, such as parsley, crushed red pepper, green chiles, chopped tomato, or basil. Take container with you to work. Put in the lunchroom refrigerator.

2. On your morning break, microwave eggs using the following timing suggestions. Stir once halfway through the cooking process.

    1 egg: 30 to 45 seconds

    2 eggs: 1 to 1½ minutes

    4 eggs: 2½ to 3 minutes

    6 eggs: 3½ to 4½ minutes

3. Eat eggs with a fork you keep in your desk. Enjoy fruit.

Meat, Cheese, and Vegetable Rollups

A balanced breakfast that tastes like a deli sandwich.

6 large lettuce leaves

6 (½ oz.) slices deli meats of your choice: lean roast beef, ham, or turkey

2 tsp. mayonnaise

½ tsp. Dijon mustard

6 (½ oz.) slices deli cheese of your choice, Swiss, cheddar, or Monterey Jack

6 apple wedges or small sweet pickles

Place lettuce leaves on the working area. Top each with one slice meat. Spread with mayo and mustard. Top with one slice cheese and one apple wedge or pickle. Roll up and secure with a toothpick.

Yields 6 rollups
Prep time: 5 minutes
Cook time: none
Serving size: 3 rollups
Each serving:
Glycemic index: low
Glycemic load: 5
Calories: 332
Protein: 21 grams
Carbohydrates: 17 grams
Fiber: 2 grams
Fat: 20 grams
Saturated fat: 10 grams

Black Bean Breakfast Salad

A high-protein vegetarian powerhouse of marinated beans and rice with cottage cheese flavored with a red wine vinegar and olive oil vinaigrette dressing.

1 (15-oz.) can black beans, drained—about 1¾ cups

1 cup cooked basmati rice

1 cup chopped fresh tomato

1 cup shredded carrots

1 green onion, sliced

2 TB. red wine vinegar

2 TB. olive oil

½ tsp. salt

¼ tsp. ground black pepper

1 cup 2 percent cottage cheese

Yields 5 cups
Prep time: 15 minutes
Cook time: none
Serving size: 1 cup salad
Each serving:
Glycemic index: low
Glycemic load: 8
Calories: 210
Protein: 13 grams
Carbohydrates: 25 grams
Fiber: 6 grams
Fat: 6.5 grams
Saturated fat: 1.26 grams

1. In a mixing bowl, stir together beans, rice, tomato, carrots, green onion, red wine vinegar, olive oil, salt, and pepper. Let stand for 5–10 minutes to let flavors blend.

2. Stir in cottage cheese. Serve.

3. This breakfast salad can be stored in an airtight storage bowl in the refrigerator.

High-Protein Blueberry Smoothie

Yields 2 cups
Prep time: 5 minutes
Cook time: none
Serving size: 2 cups smoothie
Each serving:
Glycemic index: low
Glycemic load: 10
Calories: 234
Protein: 23 grams
Carbohydrates: 33 grams
Fiber: 1 gram
Fat: 1.1 grams
Saturated fat: .70 grams

The creamy, slightly tangy taste of yogurt blended with cottage cheese and blueberries delivers high nutrition for a quick high-protein breakfast.

¾ **cup nonfat plain yogurt**

1 **cup fresh or frozen blueberries**

2 **TB. whey protein powder**

¼ **cup 2 percent cottage cheese**

¼ **tsp. stevia with FOS**

½ **tsp. vanilla extract**

Place yogurt, blueberries, whey protein powder, cottage cheese, stevia, and vanilla extract in a blender and blend until smooth. Serve cold.

Tasty Tidbits

Perhaps your mother never said, "Eat your blueberries," but she could have. Blueberries are higher in antioxidants than most other fruit and provide nutritional support for all body functions, including mental processing.

Peaches and Milk Breakfast Shake

Yields 3½ cups
Prep time: 3 minutes
Cook time: none
Serving size: 3½ cups shake
Each serving:
Glycemic index: low
Glycemic load: 12
Calories: 337
Protein: 22 grams
Carbohydrates: 52 grams
Fiber: 6 grams
Fat: 4.5 grams
Saturated fat: 2.3

Sliced peaches are combined with milk, cottage cheese, and sweet spices to add a great start to your morning.

½ **cup low-fat milk**

½ **cup 2 percent cottage cheese**

1 **cup sliced peaches**

3 **TB. wheat germ**

⅛ **tsp. nutmeg**

⅛ **tsp. cinnamon**

1½ **cups ice**

1. Pour milk and cottage cheese into a blender. Add peaches, wheat germ, and spices.

2. Blend for 30 seconds, adding ice slowly. Continue blending until shake is smooth and icy.

Cheese, Crackers, and Fruit Breakfast

Tastes like a picnic with sharp cheddar and sweet fruit.

2 oz. low-fat (2 grams fat/oz.) sharp cheddar cheese, or your choice

2 low-fat, rye Crispbread crackers

1 piece fruit, such as apple, pear, orange, bunch grapes

Eat cheese with crackers and fruit.

Yields 2 oz. cheese and fruit
Prep time: 5 minutes
Cook time: none
Serving size: full recipe
Each serving:
Glycemic index: low
Glycemic load: 20
Calories: 293
Protein: 17 grams
Carbohydrates: 45 grams
Fiber: 5 grams
Fat: 5 grams
Saturated fat: 2.4 grams

Cream Cheese Breakfast

Celery stuffed with flavored cream cheese.

1 oz. cream cheese, plain or your choice of flavors

1 oz. brick or cheddar cheese

2 ribs celery, washed and trimmed

1 piece fresh ripe fruit, such as apple, pear, orange

Fill celery ribs with cream cheese. Eat at home or pack along with fresh ripe fruit.

Variation: For lower fat and lower saturated fat, use low-fat cream cheese and 4 walnut halves. Results: 257 calories, 10.8 grams fat, 3.8 grams saturated fat.

Yields 2 celery stalks with cheese and 1 piece fruit
Prep time: 5 minutes
Serving size: full recipe
Each serving:
Glycemic index: low
Glycemic load: 12
Calories: 272
Protein: 10 grams
Carbohydrates: 30 grams
Fiber: 3 grams
Fat: 12.5 grams
Saturated fat: 7.8 grams

Home-Cooked Goodness

You obtain 2 to 3 of your 5 to 10 daily servings of vegetables and fruit with this breakfast, and enough protein to hold you until lunch.

Coconut Oatmeal Cinnamon Granola

Yields 22 cups
Prep time: 15 minutes
Cook time: 45 minutes
Serving size: ½ cup gra- nola
Each serving:
Glycemic index: low
Glycemic load: 12
Calories: 234
Protein: 6 grams
Carbohydrates: 30 grams
Fiber: 2 grams
Fat: 10 grams
Saturated fat: 1.68 grams

Granola flavored with cinnamon and honey is sweet and crunchy. Makes a large batch so you can store in the refrigerator and enjoy for breakfast over several weeks.

12 cups long-cooking oatmeal

1 cup shredded coconut

1 cup unsalted sunflower seeds

1½ cups unsalted cashews

1½ cups chopped walnuts

⅔ cups sesame seeds

½ cup canola oil

1 cup pure honey

⅔ cup water

1 TB. cinnamon

1 TB. vanilla

4 cups raisins

1. Preheat the oven to 325°F.

2. Mix oatmeal, coconut, sunflower seeds, cashews, walnuts, and sesame seeds in a large bowl.

3. In a small bowl, stir together oil, honey, water, cinnamon, and vanilla. Pour over dry ingredients and stir well.

4. Spread mixture on 2 large baking pans with sides. Bake at 325°F for 45 minutes, or until mixture is golden brown. Stir frequently. Cool.

5. Add raisins. Store in a tightly covered container in the refrigerator.

 Glycemic Notes

Granola provides carbohydrates, good fats, and high fiber for top-of-the-morning nutritional goodness. Because it's not low-glycemic, keep your portion sizes small to manage your daily glycemic load.

Chapter 4

Leisurely Breakfasts and Brunch

In This Chapter

◆ The delights of leisurely morning eating

◆ Scrumptious low-glycemic recipes

◆ Using farm-sourced ingredients

Relaxed, slow breakfasts seem like a reward—just desserts for working so hard the rest of the week. Brunch is your time to kick back and enjoy the goodness of your life and the bounty of your kitchen.

Our recipes give you *nutrient-dense* meals that are mostly low glycemic. Nutrient-dense means a food contains the most nutrients—vitamins, minerals, antioxidants—and food value possible in every bite. When you eat more nutrient-dense foods, you meet more of your daily basic nutrient needs and your hunger is more satisfied while consuming less. Nutrient-dense foods are the opposite of empty-calorie foods. As you'll see when you read through this chapter, some of the recipes are medium glycemic, like the blintzes.

Lemon Chicken Crustless Quiche

Yields 1 quiche
Prep time: 20 minutes
Cook time: 35 minutes
Serving size: ⅙ quiche
Each serving:
Glycemic index: very low
Glycemic load: 0
Calories: 192
Protein: 21 grams
Carbohydrates: <1 gram
Fiber: <1 gram
Fat: 12 grams
Saturated fat: 7 grams

Chicken is combined with the flavors of watercress, lemon, and mild cheddar cheese for a creamy breakfast quiche.

1 onion, chopped	2 eggs, lightly beaten
1 tsp. minced garlic	¼ cup heavy cream
1 TB. olive oil	3 TB. plain yogurt
2 cups chopped cooked chicken	¼ tsp. nutmeg
	1 tsp. caraway seeds
¼ cup chopped watercress leaves	3 TB. grated mild cheddar cheese
2 tsp. dried lemon peel	Salt and black pepper

1. Preheat the oven to 350°F.

2. Sauté onion and garlic in oil until softened. Remove from heat.

3. Mix onion, chicken, watercress, and lemon peel. Place in oiled baking pan or 10-inch pie pan. Beat together eggs, cream, yogurt, nutmeg, caraway seeds, cheese, salt, and pepper. Pour over chicken mixture.

4. Bake for 35 minutes or until golden.

Variation: For lower fat, use 1 egg and 2 egg whites, substitute low-fat yogurt for the heavy cream. Use low-fat yogurt, and low-fat cheddar cheese. Results: 142 calories, 6 grams fat, 2 grams saturated fat.

Tasty Tidbits

This quiche calls for mild cheese so you don't overwhelm the subtler flavors of chicken and watercress.

Baked Chile Relleno Eggs

These eggs are a show stopper—they'll win applause with the first bite. Creamy cheese and eggs are spiced up with green chiles.

2 (4-oz.) cans whole green chiles, or 8 fresh roasted

2 cups grated Monterey Jack cheese, divided

1½ TB. butter

6 eggs

1 TB. flour

2 cups milk

⅛ tsp. chili powder

Yields 1 soufflé	
Prep time: 10 minutes	
Cook time: 45 minutes to 1 hour	
Serving size: ⅙ soufflé	
Each serving:	
Glycemic index: low	
Glycemic load: 2	
Calories: 282	
Protein: 18 grams	
Carbohydrates: 5 grams	
Fiber: <1 gram	
Fat: 21 grams	
Saturated fat: 12 grams	

1. Preheat the oven to 325°F.

2. Slit each chile down one side and fill loosely with grated cheese, using one cup cheese for all chiles. Lay filled chiles in a lightly buttered, soufflé-type baking dish.

3. In a separate bowl, beat eggs and flour. Stir in milk and chili powder. Fold in remaining grated cheese.

4. Pour egg mixture over chiles. Bake for 45 minutes to 1 hour, until top is bubbly and a knife inserted near center comes out clean.

Variation: For lower fat, use low-fat cheese, 2 percent milk, and substitute olive oil for butter, and 3 eggs and 5 egg whites for the six eggs. Results: 218 calories, 14 grams fat, 6 grams saturated fat.

For even lower-fat option, use fat-free cheese. Results: 155 calories, 7 grams fat 7, 2 grams saturated fat.

Tasty Tidbits

This is a perfect breakfast soufflé—It probably won't fall, but if it does, you won't care, because it tastes great anyway. Serve with fresh fruit. Save leftovers for a quick cold breakfast or two, later in the week.

Breakfast Burritos with Sausage

Yields 8 burritos
Prep time: 10 minutes
Cook time: 20 minutes
Serving size: 1 burrito
Each serving:
Glycemic index: low
Glycemic load: 16
Calories: 390
Protein: 35 grams
Carbohydrates: 31 grams
Fiber: 4 grams
Fat: 12 grams
Saturated fat: 5 grams

The sausage, cheese, and eggs bring a hearty and savory flavor to your breakfast table.

1½ lbs. ground seasoned low-fat sausage (93% lean, 2 grams fat/oz.)

1 onion, diced

½ green pepper, diced

1 (4.5-oz.) can chopped green chiles

5 tomatoes, diced

10 eggs, beaten

1 cup shredded cheddar cheese, divided

8 flour tortillas

1 cup salsa

1. Fry sausage in a skillet until browned. Remove sausages, drain skillet, and press fat from sausages with paper towels.

2. Return sausages to the skillet and add onion, green pepper, and chiles. Sauté until tender.

3. Add tomatoes. Pour eggs and cheese on top, and stir until lightly scrambled. Fill warmed tortillas with egg mixture. Serve with salsa.

Variation: For lower fat, use 3 whole eggs and 14 egg whites and low-fat cheese. Results: 354 calories, 10 grams fat, 4 grams saturated fat.

Tasty Tidbits

Lower the glycemic value of this recipe by eating the filling without a tortilla.

Cheese and Cherry Blintzes

Tastes like a luscious dessert with vanilla, sweet cherries, and almond flavor.

8 oz. 2 percent cottage cheese

½ tsp. salt

1 egg, well beaten

½ tsp. vanilla

¼ cup dried cherries

¼ cup sliced almonds

¾ cup water or skim milk

2 eggs, well beaten

1 cup sifted flour

¼ tsp. salt

2 tsp. olive oil

Yields 8 blintzes
Prep time: 15 minutes
Cook time: 15 minutes
Serving size: 2 blintzes
Each serving:
Glycemic index: medium
Glycemic load: 23
Calories: 286
Protein: 14 grams
Carbohydrates: 35 grams
Fiber: 1 gram
Fat: 10 grams
Saturated fat: 2 grams

1. In a small bowl, prepare filling. Mix cottage cheese with salt, egg, vanilla, dried cherries, and almonds.

2. To prepare batter, stir milk into beaten eggs and gradually fold in flour and salt. Beat until smooth.

3. Heat olive oil in a 7-inch skillet over medium heat. Pour enough batter into the hot pan to just cover bottom. As soon as edges of pancake begin to curl away from sides of the pan, turn out onto wax paper and spread with a spoonful of cheese filling. Fold sides over to make a neat package.

4. Make additional blintzes with remaining batter and filling.

5. Place blintzes on a hot buttered frying pan and cook until browned. Turn and cook on other side. Serve at once.

Variation: Substitute chopped dried apricots, raisins, or chopped dates for the cherries in this recipe. You can also substitute chopped walnuts or pecans for the almonds.

Crab and Egg Bake

Yields 1 10-inch quiche
Prep time: 15 minutes
Cook time: 45 minutes
Serving size: ¹/₆ quiche
Each serving:
Glycemic index: low
Glycemic load: 3
Calories: 344
Protein: 24 grams
Carbohydrates: 8 grams
Fiber: <1 gram
Fat: 24 grams
Saturated fat: 11 grams

A very creamy, rich quiche with crabmeat and Swiss cheese delicately flavored with nutmeg.

4 eggs

1½ cups sour cream

½ cup grated Parmesan cheese

¼ cup flour

⅛ tsp. salt

4 drops Tabasco sauce

1 (6.5-oz.) can crabmeat, drained

2 cups grated Swiss cheese

1 cup chopped fresh mushrooms

1 green onion, minced

2 TB. butter

¼ tsp. nutmeg

1. Preheat the oven to 350°F.

2. Combine eggs, sour cream, Parmesan cheese, flour, salt, and Tabasco sauce in a large bowl. Beat with a whisk until smooth. Stir in crabmeat and Swiss cheese.

3. Sauté mushrooms and green onion in butter until soft and add to mixture. Stir in nutmeg.

4. Pour into an ungreased 10-inch pie or quiche pan. Bake for 45 minutes or until a knife inserted near center comes out clean. Cool 5 minutes before serving.

Variation: For lower fat, use no-fat sour cream, low-fat Swiss cheese, and use olive oil for butter. Results: 200 calories, 8 grams fat, 3 grams saturated fat.

Eggs with Tomatoes and Potatoes

This large breakfast omelet contains hash browns, tomatoes, chiles, and cheese for a mildly spicy, creamy flavor.

1 tsp. olive oil

1 (20-oz.) pkg. frozen hash brown potatoes (3½ cups)

¼ tsp. salt

1 large onion, chopped

1 TB. olive oil

2 (14.5-oz.) cans diced tomatoes with green chiles, undrained

1 (4.25-oz.) can chopped black olives

¼ tsp. ground black pepper

8 eggs

⅓ cup 2% milk

1 cup shredded Monterey Jack cheese blend

Yields 1 (9×13) omelet
Prep time: 25 minutes
Cook time: 30–35 minutes
Serving size: ⅑ pan
Each serving:
Glycemic index: low
Glycemic load: 5
Calories: 195
Protein: 12 grams
Carbohydrates: 12 grams
Fiber: 1 gram
Fat: 11 grams
Saturated fat: 4 grams

1. Preheat the oven to 375°F.

2. Lightly coat a 9×13-inch baking dish with olive oil. Place potatoes evenly in dish; sprinkle with ¼ teaspoon salt. Set aside.

3. In a large skillet over medium heat, cook onion in oil until tender. Add undrained tomatoes, olives, and pepper. Bring to boil; reduce heat. Lower heat, simmer, uncovered, for 10 minutes, stirring occasionally. Spoon over potatoes in dish.

4. In a large mixing bowl, whisk together eggs and milk; pour evenly over mixture in dish. Sprinkle with cheese.

5. Bake, uncovered, for 30–35 minutes or until set.

Polenta with Eggs

Yields 3 eggs plus polenta
Prep time: 15 minutes
Cook time: 35 minutes
Serving size: 1 egg plus ¼ cup polenta
Each serving:
Glycemic index: medium
Glycemic load: 16
Calories: 332
Protein: 20 grams
Carbohydrates: 27 grams
Fiber: 2 grams
Fat: 16 grams
Saturated fat: 6 grams

Polenta serves as a base for crispy prosciutto, eggs, and Italian cheese.

2 tsp. olive oil

8 thin slices prosciutto

3 cups water

1 tsp. salt

1 cup coarsely ground polenta

1 cup 2 percent milk

4 large eggs

¼ cup grated pecorino or Romano cheese

1. In a large frying pan over medium heat, heat olive oil. Add prosciutto slices, turning once until slices are crisp at the edges. Remove from heat to a plate and keep warm.

2. In a large, heavy saucepan over high heat, bring water and salt to a boil. Gradually stir polenta mixture into boiling water. Add milk. Stir constantly and bring to boil.

3. Reduce heat to medium-low and cook, stirring frequently, until polenta is thick and creamy, about 25 minutes. Add additional small amounts of water if polenta begins to stick.

4. Cook eggs in a skillet to your preference: poached, fried, sunny-side up.

5. Divide polenta among 4 individual plates. Top with 2 prosciutto slices. Top with an egg and sprinkle with 2 tablespoons pecorino cheese.

 Tasty Tidbits

Pecorino is a modern Italian cheese with a mild flavor. You can substitute another cheese such as Romano if your grocer doesn't stock pecorino.

Fried Eggs with Asparagus and Salami

Enjoy the complex tastes of asparagus, salami, and Parmesan cheese with your morning egg.

16 asparagus spears, trimmed

4 thin round salami slices

1 TB. olive oil

4 large eggs

4 tsp. shredded Parmesan cheese

Yields 4 eggs plus asparagus and salami
Prep time: 10 minutes
Cook time: 25 minutes
Serving size: 1 egg, plus 3 asparagus spears and 1 slice salami
Each serving:
Glycemic index: very low
Glycemic load: 0
Calories: 182
Protein: 12 grams
Carbohydrates: 2 grams
Fiber: 1 gram
Fat: 14 grams
Saturated fat: 4 grams

1. In a saucepan fitted with a vegetable steamer over boiling water, steam asparagus until just tender, about 3–5 minutes.

2. In a skillet over medium-high heat, fry salami until lightly browned. Remove and drain on paper towels to remove excess fat.

3. Wipe pan with towels to remove fat. Return to heat.

4. Heat olive oil. Break eggs into the pan. Reduce heat to low. Cook until egg whites are set and yolks begin to firm around the edges, 5–7 minutes. Remove from heat.

5. Prepare individual serving plates. Place 3 asparagus spears on plate. Add an egg to each plate. Crumble 1 salami slice over egg and asparagus.

6. Sprinkle with 1 teaspoon Parmesan cheese.

Variation: You can substitute bacon or Italian pancetta for the salami in this recipe.

 Glycemic Notes

Be sure to purchase freshly shredded Parmesan cheese and not the kind that comes in a box or shaker. The flavor of fresh Parmesan adds more zing and flavor to your meal. The boxed versions taste bland and wooden.

Frittata with Spinach, Bacon, and Swiss Cheese

Yields 1 frittata
Prep time: 15 minutes
Cook time: 15 minutes
Serving size: 1 frittata wedge
Each serving:
Glycemic index: very low
Glycemic load: 0
Calories: 147
Protein: 11 grams
Carbohydrates: 1 gram
Fiber: <1 gram
Fat: 11 grams
Saturated fat: 5 grams

A creamy, hearty frittata that's filled with the French-inspired ingredient combination of spinach, bacon, and Swiss cheese.

2 TB. olive oil

½ cup chopped green onion

¼ tsp. salt

⅛ tsp. freshly ground black pepper

6 large eggs

4 cups fresh spinach, torn into bite-size pieces

2 TB. chopped fresh parsley

2 TB. crumbled bacon

¼ cup shredded low-fat Swiss cheese

1. In a skillet, melt olive oil over medium heat. Add green onions, season with salt and pepper, and cook, stirring for about 10 minutes or until softened.

2. In a bowl, whisk eggs. Add spinach, parsley, bacon, and cheese. Pour egg mixture into the skillet and stir.

3. Reduce heat to low and cook until eggs are set around the edges, but still a little moist in the center, about 15 minutes. Turn frittata. Cook until eggs are set.

4. Cut into 6 wedges and serve.

Hazelnut Sour Cream Pancakes

Sour cream lends a tangy touch to these wholesome crunchy pancakes.

¾ cup stone-ground whole-wheat flour

½ cup Hi-Maize Resistant Starch

¾ cup finely chopped hazelnuts

2 TB. honey

1 TB. baking powder

½ tsp. salt

1¼ cups milk

2 eggs, lightly beaten

1 (8-oz.) carton sour cream

2 TB. canola oil

Yields 16 pancakes
Prep time: 15 minutes
Cook time: 2 minutes per batch
Serving size: 2 pancakes
Each serving:
Glycemic index: low
Glycemic load: 7
Calories: 278
Protein: 8 grams
Carbohydrates: 21 grams
Fiber: 3 grams
Fat: 18 grams
Saturated fat: 7 grams

1. In a large bowl, combine flour, Hi-Maize, hazelnuts, honey, baking powder, and salt. In second bowl, combine milk, eggs, sour cream, and oil. Stir milk mixture into flour mixture until slightly lumpy.

2. Heat a lightly oiled griddle or heavy skillet over medium heat. For each pancake, pour ¼ cup batter onto the griddle. Cook until golden; turn when tops are bubbly and edges are slightly dry (1–2 minutes per side).

Variation: For lower fat, use skim milk and low-fat sour cream. Results: 242 calories, 14 grams fat, 4 grams saturated fat. You can also substitute walnuts or pine nuts for the hazelnuts.

Pancakes with Pumpkin and Spices

Yields 16 pancakes
Prep time: 10 minutes
Cook time: 2 minutes per batch
Serving size: 2 pancakes
Each serving:
Glycemic index: low
Glycemic load: 14
Calories: 204
Protein: 7 grams
Carbohydrates: 26 grams
Fiber: 2 grams
Fat: 8 grams
Saturated fat: 2 grams

Cook up a batch in cold weather and near the holidays. Tastes like pumpkin pie seasoned with cinnamon and cloves.

1 cup stone-ground whole-wheat flour

1 cup Hi-Maize Resistant Starch

3 TB. honey

1 TB. baking powder

½ tsp. salt

1½ cups milk

3 eggs, lightly beaten

1 cup canned pumpkin

½ tsp. cinnamon

¼ tsp. ground cloves

3 TB. canola oil

1. In a large bowl, combine flour, Hi-Maize, honey, baking powder, and salt. In a second bowl, combine milk, eggs, pumpkin, cinnamon, cloves, and oil. Stir milk mixture into flour mixture until slightly lumpy.

2. Heat a lightly greased griddle or skillet over medium heat. For each pancake, pour ¼ cup batter onto griddle. Cook until golden; turn when tops are bubbly and edges are slightly dry.

Pecan-Crusted French Toast

The rich, sweet batter is flavored with cinnamon and vanilla.

4 eggs, beaten lightly

1 cup milk

2 tsp. honey

½ cup chopped pecans

¼ tsp. salt

1 tsp. cinnamon

1 tsp. vanilla

2 TB. canola oil

4 slices stone-ground whole-wheat bread

Yields 4 slices toast
Prep time: 10 minutes
Cook time: 10 minutes
Serving size: 1 slice toast
Each serving:
Glycemic index: low
Glycemic load: 10
Calories: 310
Protein: 16 grams
Carbohydrates: 21 grams
Fiber: 6 grams
Fat: 18 grams
Saturated fat: 3 grams

1. In a mixing bowl, add eggs, milk, honey, pecans, salt, cinnamon, and vanilla.

2. Heat oil in large skillet over medium-high heat. Dip whole-wheat bread in egg mixture. Add dipped bread to the skillet. Pour remaining batter over bread. Cook until bottom of bread is toasted. Turn and cook until egg mixture is cooked and bottom is lightly browned.

Home-Cooked Goodness

As you cook the toast, it will look like an omelet with bread in it. This adds to the custardy taste of the toast and increases the protein content.

Overnight Oatmeal

Rich and hearty oatmeal with vanilla, cranberries, and almonds.

Yields 4 cups oatmeal
Prep time: overnight
Cook time: 15 minutes evening, 5 minutes in morning
Serving size: 1 cup oatmeal
Each serving:
Glycemic index: low
Glycemic load: 12
Calories: 210
Protein: 9 grams
Carbohydrates: 30 grams
Fiber: 5 grams
Fat: 6 grams
Saturated fat: 0.25 grams

4 cups water

1 cup steel-cut oats, not long-cooking or quick oatmeal

1 tsp. vanilla

½ cup dried cranberries

½ cup slivered almonds

1. The evening before, in a saucepan, bring water to a boil over high heat. Add oatmeal. Stir until all the liquid has been absorbed. Turn off the heat, cover the pot, and leave overnight.

2. In the morning, bring oats to a brisk boil over high heat and cook until just tender. Stir in vanilla, cranberries, and almonds.

Home-Cooked Goodness

Prepare steel-cut oatmeal the evening before to shorten morning preparation time. Vary fruit and nut additions with chopped dates, dried or fresh blueberries, raisins, pecans, walnuts, or pine nuts. Serve with eggs or cheese for a balanced meal.

Breads

In This Chapter

- ◆ Breads for eating low glycemic
- ◆ Yeast breads and quick breads
- ◆ Crackers for appetizers and snacks

Bake the bread recipes in this chapter and you'll enjoy the comforting and friendly taste of bread in a new way. The recipes you'll find here are low or medium glycemic and the breads are good for your waistline and your health.

Because white and finely milled flour is high glycemic, we've used some lower-glycemic ingredients, such as oat bran, rye flour, Hi-Maize Resistant Starch, and stone-ground whole-wheat flour. Sourdough bread is lower glycemic because it's naturally sour, and we've used whole-wheat flour in that recipe.

You'll find recipes for yeast breads, quick breads, crackers, rolls, and biscuits, with plenty of variations to give you a wide array of tastes to choose from.

Cornbread with Bacon and Cheese

A savory cornbread with cheddar cheese and crumbled bacon.

Yields 1 (9-inch) pan
Prep time: 20 minutes
Cook time: 40–45 minutes
Serving size: 1 wedge corn bread, 2³/₄ inches at wide edge
Each serving:
Glycemic index: low
Glycemic load: 11
Calories: 236
Protein: 11 grams
Carbohydrates: 21 grams
Fiber: 3 grams
Fat: 12 grams
Saturated fat: 4 grams

1 cup coarse yellow cornmeal

½ cup Hi-Maize Resistant Starch

½ cup oat bran

½ tsp. baking soda

½ tsp. salt

1 cup milk

2 eggs

2 TB. olive oil

1 cup cheddar cheese, grated

1 onion, chopped

12 slices bacon, cooked, drained, and crumbled

2 TB. pimentos, chopped

1. Preheat the oven to 350°F.

2. Whisk together cornmeal, Hi-Maize, oat bran, baking soda, and salt. Add milk, eggs, and olive oil. Stir well.

3. Fold in cheddar cheese, onion, bacon, and pimentos.

4. Pour into an oiled 9-inch round baking dish. Bake for 40–45 minutes.

Crisp Rosemary Flatbread

A rosemary-flavored cracker that's great for cheeses and spreads.

Yields 1 (9×13-inch) pan
Prep time: 5 minutes
Cook time: 20 minutes plus 30–40 minutes rest time
Serving size: 1 (4.5× 3-inch) cracker
Each serving:
Glycemic index: low
Glycemic load: 6
Calories: 122
Protein: 7 grams
Carbohydrates: 18 grams
Fiber: 7 grams
Fat: 2.5 grams
Saturated fat: 1 grams

4 eggs

1²/₃ cups wheat bran

1¹/₃ cups thick-cut oats

1 tsp. dried rosemary, crumbled

1 tsp. baking powder

1 TB. xylitol

1. Preheat the oven to 325°F.

2. In a mixing bowl, beat eggs until fluffy. Stir in wheat bran, oats, rosemary, baking powder, and xylitol. Flatten dough and press onto a 9×13-inch baking dish.

3. Bake for 20 minutes. Turn off oven and let bread stay in oven for an additional 30–40 minutes.

Sweet Potato Biscuits

Sweet potato biscuits accented with cinnamon.

1 egg
⅓ cup butter
1 cup cooked, mashed sweet potatoes
2 TB. honey

½ cup stone-ground whole-wheat flour
½ cup oat bran
2 tsp. baking powder
½ tsp. cinnamon
½ tsp. salt

Yields 12 biscuits
Prep time: 10 minutes
Cook time: 10–20 minutes
Serving size: 1 biscuit
Each serving:
Glycemic index: low
Glycemic load: 6
Calories: 110
Protein: 3 grams
Carbohydrates: 11 grams
Fiber: 2 grams
Fat: 6 grams
Saturated fat: 2 grams

1. Preheat the oven to 375°F.

2. In an electric mixer, beat egg, butter, sweet potatoes, and honey until fluffy. Add flour, oat bran, baking powder, and salt. Blend well and drop by tablespoons onto a lightly greased baking pan.

3. Bake 10–20 minutes. Check after 10 minutes—biscuits will be done when they're an even light brown.

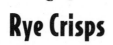

Rye Crisps

Buttery rye crackers flavored with caraway seeds.

2 cups whole-grain dark rye flour
1 cup whole-wheat flour
1 cup oat bran
½ tsp. salt

¼ tsp. baking soda
¼ cup butter, melted
¼ cup olive oil
1 cup (or more) water
1 tsp. caraway seeds

Yields 36 crackers
Prep time: 10 minutes
Cook time: 30 minutes
Serving size: 3 crackers
Each serving:
Glycemic index: low
Glycemic load: 14
Calories: 188
Protein: 5 grams
Carbohydrates: 27 grams
Fiber: 5 grams
Fat: 8 grams
Saturated fat: 1 gram

1. Preheat the oven to 275°F.

2. In a mixing bowl, combine rye flour, wheat flour, oat bran, salt, baking soda, butter, olive oil, water, and caraway seeds. Stir to mix well. If dough is too stiff and won't form a stiff ball, add water in increments of 1 tablespoon until dough is barely pliable.

3. Roll out dough thinly on floured surface. Cut into desired shapes. Bake on cookie sheets for about 30 minutes.

Variation: Use poppy seeds in place of caraway seeds.

Berry Cornbread Loaves

Cornbread with the sweet fruit flavors of berries and orange.

Yields 5 loaves
Prep time: 25 minutes
Cook time: 18 minutes
Serving size: 1 (1-inch) slice bread
Each serving:
Glycemic index: low
Glycemic load: 5
Calories: 78
Protein: 2 grams
Carbohydrates: 12 grams
Fiber: 2 grams
Fat: 2.5 grams
Saturated fat: <1 grams

½ cup yellow cornmeal

½ cup flour

½ cup oat bran

½ cup Hi-Maize Resistant Starch

½ cup xylitol

2 tsp. baking powder

¼ tsp. salt

⅔ cup skim milk

2 TB. butter, melted

2 TB. olive oil

2 large eggs, lightly beaten

2 tsp. dried orange peel

¾ cup fresh raspberries

¾ cup fresh blueberries

1. Preheat the oven to 400°F. Line 5 (5³/₄×3×2-inch) disposable foil loaf pans with parchment paper.

2. In a large bowl, combine cornmeal, flour, oat bran, Hi-Maize, xylitol, baking powder, and salt. Add milk, butter, olive oil, eggs, and orange peel. Stir to blend. Gently stir in raspberries and blueberries. Evenly divide batter among loaf pans.

3. Bake 18–20 minutes until tops are lightly golden and a toothpick inserted in center comes out clean. Remove from the pans. Cool on a wire rack before serving.

Home-Cooked Goodness

Mini-loaves give you a terrific way to enjoy cornbread. You can serve one or two, depending on the size of your family, and freeze the rest for a meal later in the month.

Sourdough Bread and Starter

A delicious favorite that gives you fresh sourdough flavor and low-glycemic benefits.

1 pkg. dry yeast	**¼ cup canola oil**
2 cups warm water	**½ cup water**
2 cups unbleached flour	**1 tsp. salt**
1 pkg. dry yeast	**⅓ cup sugar**
¼ cup warm water	**1 cup sourdough starter**
1 tsp. sugar	**3½ cups whole-wheat flour**
1 egg	

1. Empty yeast into a warm ceramic or glass mixing bowl (not metal) and stir in water until yeast is dissolved. Add flour and stir until well blended. Cover with plastic wrap and let stand at room temperature for about 48 hours. (When ready, the starter will be bubbly with a somewhat yellowish liquid on top.)

2. Store starter in the refrigerator in a jar with a loose-fitting lid. Every time part of the starter is removed to make bread, it must be replenished. At least once a week, mix together sourdough starter, 1 cup flour, 1 cup milk, and ⅓ cup sugar. Keep 1 cup of this mixture on hand for replenishing.

3. In a mixing bowl, dissolve yeast in ¼ cup warm water, stirring in sugar. Let sit 15 minutes.

4. Mix egg, canola oil, ½ cup water, salt, and ⅓ cup sugar in a large ceramic or glass mixing bowl. Add sourdough starter and yeast mixture to egg mixture.

5. With electric mixer, blend in 2 cups flour, then add remaining flour and mix with a wooden spoon. Turn onto floured board and knead 10–20 times. Add a bit more flour if still sticky.

6. Wipe inside of bowl to clean. Oil inside of bowl. Put dough in the bowl, turning to make sure the top of dough is oiled. Cover the bowl with a cloth and let rise 2 hours in a warm place.

7. After dough has risen to double in bulk, punch down, place on the floured board, and knead again for 2 minutes. Divide into 2 balls and place in 2 well-greased (9×5-inch) bread pans. Cover and let rise 2 more hours in a warm place.

8. Bake at 350°F for 20–25 minutes.

Yields 2 loaves bread plus 3 cups starter
Prep time: 10 minutes plus 48 hours for starter (20 minutes plus 4 hours rise time for bread)
Cook time: 20–25 minutes
Serving size: ½-inch slice bread
Each serving:
Glycemic index: low
Glycemic load: 8
Calories: 86
Protein: 3 grams
Carbohydrates: 14 grams
Fiber: 2 grams
Fat: 2 grams
Saturated fat: <1 gram

Home-Cooked Goodness

Begin bread-making early enough so you can have warm bread for dinner. Store extra loaves in the freezer for later use.

Stone-Ground Whole-Wheat Bread

A scrumptious bread with a rich wheat taste.

Yields 2 loaves
Prep time: 10 minutes plus 5 hours rise time
Cook time: 40–45 minutes
Serving size: 1 (¹/₂-inch) slice bread
Each serving:
Glycemic index: medium
Glycemic load: 9
Calories: 98
Protein: 3 grams
Carbohydrates: 17 grams
Fiber: 2 grams
Fat: 2 grams
Saturated fat: <1 gram

2 TB. active dry yeast

¹/₄ cup warm water (110°F/43°C)

¹/₄ cup plus 2 TB. honey

1¹/₂ tsp. salt

3 TB. olive oil

1³/₄ cups warm water (110°F/43°C)

6 cups stone-ground whole-wheat flour

1. In a small bowl, dissolve yeast in ¹/₄ cup warm water. Allow to stand 3–5 minutes.

2. In a large bowl, combine honey, salt, olive oil, and 1³/₄ cups water. Add yeast mixture.

3. Stir in flour and mix well. Knead 10 minutes. Cover and let rise 1 hour and 45 minutes. Punch down.

4. Let rise 40–60 minutes until double in size. Punch down and let rise a third time until doubled.

5. Shape into 2 loaves and place in 2 (9×5-inch) loaf pans. Let loaves rise until doubled.

6. Preheat the oven to 350°F. Bake loaves for 40–45 minutes.

Variation: Roll loaves in sesame seeds or poppy seeds before baking.

 Glycemic Notes

Be sure to use a glass or ceramic bowl for making bread. A metal bowl will prevent the flour-yeast mixture from rising.

Parmesan Herb Dinner Rolls

Parmesan sparks up the flavor of these basil-and-oregano-accented rolls.

1 packet dry active yeast

1 TB. sugar

1 cup warm water

1 cup skim milk

2 eggs

1½ tsp. salt

2 TB. butter

1 tsp. dried basil

2 tsp. dried oregano

¼ cup Parmesan cheese, freshly grated

¾ cup Hi-Maize Resistant Starch

4 cups whole-wheat flour

1 egg white

2 TB. water

Yields 24 dinner rolls
Prep time: 20 minutes plus 1 hour 40 minutes rise time
Cook time: 40–45 minutes
Serving size: 1 roll
Each serving:
Glycemic index: medium
Glycemic load: 10
Calories: 117
Protein: 4 grams
Carbohydrates: 18 grams
Fiber: 3 grams
Fat: 2 grams
Saturated fat: 1 grams

1. In a small mixing bowl, dissolve yeast and sugar in warm water. Let stand 5 minutes.

2. In another mixing bowl, combine yeast mixture, milk, eggs, salt, butter, basil, oregano, Parmesan, Hi-Maize, and about 2 cups flour. Mix on low speed with a dough hook. Add remaining flour, ½ cup at a time.

3. When dough is blended, mix on medium speed for 8 minutes.

4. Shape dough into a ball. Lightly oil a large bowl and place dough in the bowl, turning to coat with oil. Cover with plastic wrap and let rise for 1 hour.

5. Oil 2 (9×13-inch) baking pans. Punch down dough and turn on a lightly floured surface. Divide dough into 24 pieces. Shape each piece into a round ball and place on prepared pans. Cover rolls with plastic wrap and let rise for 40 minutes.

6. Preheat the oven to 350°F. In a small bowl, lightly beat egg white with 2 tablespoons water. Brush on tops of rolls.

7. Bake for 20–25 minutes, or until golden brown.

Variation: Replace the basil, oregano, and Parmesan with ½ cup chopped fresh parsley and ⅓ cup chopped fresh chives.

Sesame Crackers

Toasted sesame seeds wrapped in yogurt-flavored oat bran and whole-wheat dough.

Yields 36 crackers
Prep time: 10 minutes
Cook time: 10 minutes
Serving size: 3 crackers
Each serving:
Glycemic index: low
Glycemic load: 8
Calories: 85
Protein: 3 grams
Carbohydrates: 14 grams
Fiber: 3 grams
Fat: 2 grams
Saturated fat: <1 grams

1 cup stone-ground whole-wheat flour

1 cup oat bran

1 tsp. salt

1½ tsp. baking powder

¼ cup yogurt

1 TB. butter

2 TB. sesame seeds

⅔ cup ice water

1. Preheat the oven to 350°F.

2. In a mixing bowl, combine whole-wheat flour, oat bran, salt, and baking powder. Cut in yogurt.

3. In a small skillet over medium heat, melt butter, add sesame seeds, and toast while stirring. Add sesame seeds and butter to flour mixture.

4. Mix in ice water and knead gently into a ball. Roll to ⅛ inch thick. Cut with knife into rectangles. Prick all over with fork. Place rectangles on a parchment-paper-lined baking sheet.

5. Bake 10 minutes until lightly browned. Cool on rack.

Variation: Substitute poppy seeds, chopped sunflower seeds, or chopped pine nuts for the sesame seeds.

Chapter 6

Take-Along Snacks

In This Chapter

- ◆ Knowing when you need a snack
- ◆ Making wise selections
- ◆ Averting emotional-eating pitfalls

When you feel that you need a snack, have a snack. Snacking is a natural, honest activity. Perhaps you've been led to think of having a snack as the same thing as having a sneak. Or as a failure. Or as a weakness. Don't you believe it for a moment.

Snacking is a natural part of human biology and behavior. The best time for a snack is when your stomach is hungry and your next meal is a ways off. Snacks help you manage your hunger so you don't sit down starving and ravenous for dinner and thus overeat.

Carrying along your snacks is an enlightened thing to do. After all, that's why stores sell those small, resealable snack bags—for your snacks. Keep snacks in your glove compartment, your desk, your briefcase, your handbag, your luggage. But at home, keep them in the kitchen so that you're forced to take a break when you eat a snack.

Peppered Beef Jerky

A tasty and chewy high-protein: a snack with virtually no fat that's flavored with coarsely ground black pepper.

Yields 2 lbs. flank steak
Prep time: 20 minutes plus overnight
Cook time: 5 hours
Serving size: 1/8 lb. or 2 oz. jerky
Each serving:
Glycemic index: very low
Glycemic load: 1
Calories: 117
Protein: 14 grams
Carbohydrates: 4 grams
Fiber: 0 grams
Fat: 5 grams
Saturated fat: 3 grams

2 lbs. flank steak, thinly sliced

½ cup soy sauce

¼ cup honey

6 cloves garlic, minced

1½ TB. fresh ginger root, grated

2 TB. coarsely ground black pepper

1 tsp. canola oil

1 tsp. Worcestershire sauce

1 tsp. onion powder

1. Partially freeze flank steak to assist in slicing.

2. To slice, use a very sharp knife to remove all visible fat and slice into 1/4-inch strips.

3. Combine soy sauce, honey, garlic, ginger root, 1 tablespoon black pepper, canola oil, Worcestershire sauce, and onion powder for the marinade.

4. Marinate steak in the refrigerator overnight.

5. Preheat the oven to 120°F. Place a sheet of aluminum foil on the bottom of your oven to catch drips. Drain meat in a colander and pat dry with paper towels. Carefully place meat slices directly on the racks. Sprinkle meat with remaining 1 tablespoon black pepper. Leave oven door open a crack to allow moisture to escape.

6. When jerky is firm and dry after about 4–6 hours, remove from oven, cool, and store in snack bags or container in the refrigerator.

Home-Cooked Goodness

Making beef jerky at home is a labor of love, and a smart one, too. Your ingredients are fresh and you'll have high-protein, very-low-fat snacks for your office or your children's snack times. Carry jerky with you when traveling to ensure you'll eat well.

Parmesan Crisps

It's hard to resist the wonderful cheesy flavor of Parmesan in these snack crackers.

4 oz. Parmesan cheese, cut into 1-inch chunks

¾ cup Hi-Maize Resistant Starch

3 TB. olive oil

1½ tsp. finely shredded lemon peel

¼ tsp. freshly ground black pepper

2 TB. cold water

¼ tsp. Kosher or sea salt

½ tsp. finely shredded lemon peel

> *Yields 48 rectangles
> (24 strips)*
>
> **Prep time:** 30 minutes
>
> **Cook time:** 10 minutes
>
> **Serving size:** 2 cracker strips
>
> **Each serving:**
> Glycemic index: low
> Glycemic load: 1
> Calories: 82
> Protein: 3 grams
> Carbohydrates: 4 grams
> Fiber: 2 grams
> Fat: 6 grams
> Saturated fat: 2 grams

1. Preheat the oven to 400°F.

2. Put 2 chunks of cheese in a food processor fitted with a chopping blade. Cover and process until cheese is almost ground. Drop in remaining cheese chunks, a few at a time, until all cheese is ground.

3. Remove the top and add Hi-Maize Resistant Starch, olive oil, 1½ teaspoon lemon peel, and pepper to food processor. With machine running, add water through feed tube. Process until mixture forms a ball.

4. Flatten cheese mixture on a sheet of parchment paper or waxed paper. Top with another sheet of paper. Use a rolling pin to roll out 12-inch square. Remove the top sheet of paper. Invert dough onto a baking sheet, then remove the second sheet. Using a sharp knife or pizza cutter, cut 2-inch rectangles or ½-inch strips. Arrange on the baking sheet 1 inch apart. Using a fork, prick dough. Sprinkle with salt and additional lemon peel.

5. Bake for 10 to 15 minutes or until golden brown; cool on the baking sheet.

Home-Cooked Goodness

Nibble on a couple of these crackers accompanied by fresh fruit, raw vegetables, or deli meats.

Apricot and Almond Trail Mix

A crunchy and nourishing, fruity-tasting snack for the trail or during a long afternoon at the office.

Yields 4½ cups mix
Prep time: 10 minutes
Cook time: 5 minutes
Serving size: ¼ cup mix
Each serving:
Glycemic index: low
Glycemic load: 5
Calories: 108
Protein: 2 grams
Carbohydrates: 16 grams
Fiber: 2 grams
Fat: 4 grams
Saturated fat: <1 gram

1 tsp. canola oil

½ tsp. sesame seeds

¼ cup sliced almonds

½ cup Kashi GOLEAN Crunch

½ cup chopped walnuts

1 cup dried apricots, chopped

1. Heat oil in a small saucepan over medium heat. Add sesame seeds. When they sizzle (about 3 seconds), remove from heat. Mix in remaining ingredients.

2. Cool and store in an airtight container or serving-size plastic snack bags.

Walnut and Banana Trail Mix

The pepper in this recipe spices up the trail mix and gives it some bite to balance the sweetness.

Yields 2 cups mix
Prep time: 10 minutes
Serving size: ¼ cup mix
Each serving:
Glycemic index: low
Glycemic load: 12
Calories: 105
Protein: 1 gram
Carbohydrates: 14 grams
Fiber: 2 grams
Fat: 5 grams
Saturated fat: <1 gram

¼ cup pecans, almonds, or peanuts

½ cup dried cranberries

¼ tsp. grated lemon zest

1 cup dried banana chips

¼ cup walnut pieces

⅛ tsp. ground white pepper

1. Toss nuts, cranberries, lemon zest, banana chips, walnuts, and white pepper in a bowl and mix well.

2. Store in an airtight container.

Variation: Substitute other dried fruits you have on hand: raisins, dried cherries, or pineapple.

Home-Cooked Goodness

Flavoring trail mix with savory, tangy, or sweet herbs and spices adds to your taste satisfaction.

Turmeric Trail Mix

The spicy yellow coating adds exotic flavor and potent antioxidants to this trail mix recipe.

1 tsp. canola oil

1 cup uncooked long-cooking oatmeal

¼ cup cashews

¼ cup peanuts

3 TB. sesame seeds

¼ tsp. salt

¼ ground turmeric

½ cup golden raisins

2 TB. dried blueberries

Yields 2½ cups mix
Prep time: 5 minutes
Cook time: 5 minutes
Serving size: ¼ cup mix
Each serving:
Glycemic index: low
Glycemic load: 8
Calories: 117
Protein: 3 grams
Carbohydrates: 15 grams
Fiber: 1 gram
Fat: 5 grams
Saturated fat: 1 gram

1. Heat oil in a small saucepan over medium-low heat. Add oatmeal, cashews, peanuts, sesame seeds, and salt.

2. Toast while stirring constantly for 5 minutes to evenly toast nuts and oatmeal. Remove from heat. Mix in turmeric, raisins, and blueberries. Cool.

3. Store in an airtight container.

New Mexican Cherry Trail Mix

Cherries add a dense, sweet flavor accented by the earthy forest taste of pine nuts and pumpkin seeds.

¾ cup almonds

¼ cup dried cherries

¼ cup raisins

¼ cup pine nuts

½ cup pumpkin seeds

¼ cup chopped dried mango slices

½ tsp. chili powder (or cayenne)

Yields 2¼ cups mix
Prep time: 5 minutes
Serving size: ¼ cup mix
Each serving:
Glycemic index: low
Glycemic load: 4
Calories: 146
Protein: 4 grams
Carbohydrates: 10 grams
Fiber: 2 grams
Fat: 10 grams
Saturated fat: 1 gram

1. Toss almonds, cherries, raisins, pine nuts, pumpkin seeds, mango, and chili powder in a bowl and mix well.

2. Store in an airtight container.

Trail Mix with Chocolate Morsels

Yields 7 cups mix
Prep time: 10 minutes
Cook time: 10 minutes
Serving size: ¹/₄ cup
Each serving:
Glycemic index: medium
Glycemic load: 11
Calories: 152
Protein: 2 grams
Carbohydrates: 18 grams
Fiber: 2 grams
Fat: 8 grams
Saturated fat: 1 gram

Dark chocolate adds an indulgent taste to this rich nut and fruit mixture, while small pretzels add crunch.

1¼ **cups pecan halves**	1¼ **cups cranberries**
1¼ **cups shelled pistachio nuts**	1¼ **cups raisins**
1½ **cups small pretzels**	1 **TB. chopped fresh orange peel**
½ **cup dark chocolate morsels**	

1. Preheat the oven to 325°F.

2. Spread nuts in a shallow baking pan. Place in the oven for 10 minutes to toast, stirring every 3 minutes. Remove and cool.

3. Combine nuts with pretzels, chocolate morsels, cranberries, raisins, and orange peel.

4. Store in an airtight container at room temperature up to 1 week. Use as a dessert mix or as a topping for ice cream or fresh fruit.

 Glycemic Notes _____

Dark chocolate is a viable snack food. It's low glycemic, with a value of 48. Once considered a decadent and indulgent food, today's healthy eaters enjoy it sparingly for its high levels of antioxidants and luscious taste.

Whole-Food Bars

Crunchy energy bars are sweetened with honey.

2 cups quick oats

¾ cup wheat bran

¼ cup wheat germ

½ cup slivered almonds

½ cup pecan halves

½ cup sesame seeds

½ cup shredded coconut

½ cup raisins

½ cup dried cranberries

3 eggs

½ cup honey

½ cup canola oil

½ tsp. salt

Yields 16 bars
Prep time: 15 minutes
Cook time: 20–25 minutes
Serving size: 1 bar
Each serving:
Glycemic index: low
Glycemic load: 15
Calories: 170
Protein: 7 grams
Carbohydrates: 29 grams
Fiber: 3 grams
Fat: 15 grams
Saturated fat: 2.9 grams

1. Preheat the oven to 350°F.

2. In a large mixing bowl, mix together oats, wheat bran, wheat germ, almonds, pecans, sesame seed, coconut, raisins, and cranberries.

3. In a small bowl, beat eggs until well mixed. Stir in honey, canola oil, and salt.

4. Pour egg mixture over dry ingredients and mix well, making sure all ingredients are moistened.

5. Turn mixture into a 9×13-inch baking dish and bake for 20 to 25 minutes.

Home-Cooked Goodness

These high-fiber bars offer healthful fruit, nuts, eggs, and seeds. You'll receive lots of energy in one or two bites.

Napa Cabbage and Shrimp Wraps

Nutty-tasting wild rice combines with shrimp and tomatoes, wrapped in Napa cabbage.

Yields 6 wraps
Prep time: 15 minutes
Serving size: 1 wrap
Each serving:
Glycemic index: low
Glycemic load: 2
Calories: 134
Protein: 11 grams
Carbohydrates: 5 grams
Fiber: 1 gram
Fat: 7.75 grams
Saturated fat: <1 gram

8 oz. cooked diced shrimp

1½ cups diced tomatoes

½ cup diced celery

1 TB. chopped parsley

¼ tsp. salt

⅛ tsp. freshly ground black pepper

½ cup cooked wild rice

¼ cup mayonnaise

6 large Napa cabbage leaves

1. Place shrimp, tomatoes, celery, parsley, salt, pepper, and wild rice in a small bowl and stir in mayonnaise.

2. Divide mixture evenly among cabbage leaves. Roll up and secure with toothpicks.

Variation: Substitute lettuce leaves for the Napa cabbage.

Tuna Tortillas

Tuna, cucumber, and avocado are rolled in spinach-flavored tortillas with seasoned rice and toasted sesame seeds.

2 cups basmati rice, cooked and cooled

2 TB. toasted sesame seeds

2 TB. white-wine vinegar

2 tsp. honey

½ tsp. salt

¼ tsp. freshly ground black pepper

¼ cup mayonnaise

4 (10-inch) spinach-flavored low-carb, low-fat flour tortillas

1 (6-oz.) pkg. tuna

1 medium avocado, halved, seeded, peeled, and sliced

2 medium cucumbers, halved lengthwise and cut into thin sticks

1 cup alfalfa sprouts

Yields 28 appetizers
Prep time: 30 minutes + chill 1 hour
Cook time: 5 minutes
Serving size: 2 appetizers
Each serving:
Glycemic index: low
Glycemic load: 6
Calories: 110
Protein: 4 grams
Carbohydrates: 10 grams
Fiber: 2 grams
Fat: 6 grams
Saturated fat: 1 gram

1. In a large bowl, combine rice and sesame seeds. In a separate bowl, combine vinegar, honey, salt, and pepper. Stir until salt is dissolved. Pour vinegar mixture over rice; toss to coat. Set aside.

2. Spread 1 tablespoon of mayonnaise mixture onto each tortilla. Top half of each tortilla with rice mixture, tuna, avocado, cucumber, and sprouts. Carefully roll each tortilla tightly, starting at the filled side. Wrap each in plastic wrap. Chill for 1 to 4 hours.

3. To serve, cut each tortilla in half.

Home-Cooked Goodness

This is a great take-along snack that also works as a packed lunch. Add an apple or piece of fruit to complete your meal.

Spicy Pecans

The spicy, salty taste makes eating just a few very satisfying.

Yields 1 cup pecans
Prep time: 5 minutes
Cook time: 15 minutes
Serving size: $^1/_8$ cup pecans
Each serving:
Glycemic index: very low
Glycemic load: 0
Calories: 108
Protein: 1 gram
Carbohydrates: 2 grams
Fiber: 1 gram
Fat: 10.7 grams
Saturated fat: 1 gram

1 cup pecan halves

¼ tsp. salt

⅛ tsp. cayenne

⅛ tsp. cumin

1 TB. butter, melted (more, if using more nuts)

1. Preheat the oven to 350°F.

2. Combine nuts, salt, cayenne, cumin, and butter. Mix well.

3. Spread on a baking sheet. Bake 15 minutes, stirring once. Cool.

Home-Cooked Goodness

Any kind of nuts can be seasoned by baking as recommended in this recipe. You can also sauté nuts in a frying pan until toasty, or heat in the microwave for 45 seconds, then stir, repeating until toasty but not burned.

Part  3

On the Light Side

Enjoy satisfying lighter fare for lunches and appetizers and even late-evening snacks. You'll eat enough food to replenish your energy and keep it high until your main meal of the day.

Sauces and condiments enhance the flavors of cold cuts, meats, and undressed vegetables. Use these to vary the tastes of your meals.

Soup can be a main course or a starter, depending on your appetite preference. We give you plenty of choices.

Chapter 7

Lunches

In This Chapter

- ◆ The importance of lunch
- ◆ Eating a high-energy lunch
- ◆ Preparing lunches for home, work, and play

The recipes in this chapter give you superb choices for low-glycemic and farm-sourced lunches, which can be difficult to find at convenience stores, food carts, and vending machines. Our recipes call for cheeses, meats, freah vegetables, and fruit. They're seasoned with such condiments to fit your tastes—savory or mild.

Beef and Cabbage Wraps

The seasoned ground beef, corn, and crisp cabbage are wrapped in corn tortillas and topped with an Italian dressing.

Yields 12 (6-inch) tortillas with filling	

Prep time: 10 minutes

Cook time: 20 minutes

Serving size: 2 (6-inch) tortillas with filling

Each serving:

Glycemic index: low

Glycemic load: 13

Calories: 261

Protein: 18 grams

Carbohydrates: 28 grams

Fiber: 4 grams

Fat: 8.55 grams

Saturated fat: 1.75 grams

12 (6-inch) corn tortillas	**1 cup frozen whole-kernel corn**
12 oz. extra lean ground beef or low-fat turkey	**½ cup Italian salad dressing**
½ cup chopped onion (1 medium)	**2 cups shredded cabbage**

1. Wrap tortillas in a clean kitchen towel. Place in a microwave oven and cook on high for 1 minute. Keep wrapped until step 3. Or wrap tortillas in aluminum foil and place in oven at 350 degrees for 10 minutes.

2. In a large skillet over medium heat, cook beef and onion for 5 minutes or until beef is brown and onion is tender. Drain. Stir in corn and ¼ cup salad dressing. Cook and stir for 10 minutes or until heated through.

3. To serve, spoon about ⅓ cup filling onto each tortilla. Top with shredded cabbage and rest of salad dressing, equally dividing among tortillas. Roll to make wraps.

Tasty Tidbits

The raw cabbage in these wraps gives freshness to the classic corn tortilla. To lower the glycemic value of the wraps, substitute cabbage leaves for the corn tortillas.

Avocado and Yogurt Sandwich Spread

Here, creamy avocado, cream cheese, and yogurt are paired with southwestern spices and lime or lemon juice.

1½ cups plain low-fat yogurt

1 (8-oz.) pkg. low-fat cream cheese, softened

1 ripe avocado, halved, seeded, peeled, and diced

2 green onions, chopped

1 clove garlic, quartered

2 tsp. ground cumin

2 tsp. fresh lemon juice or lime juice

¼ tsp. bottled hot pepper sauce

⅛ tsp. ground chili powder

½ tsp. salt

½ cup snipped fresh cilantro

60 Jicama or zucchini slices

Yields 3 cups spread
Prep time: 20 minutes, plus chill overnight
Serving size: ¼ cup spread
Each serving:
Glycemic index: low
Glycemic load: 1
Calories: 71
Protein: 3.5 grams
Carbohydrates: 3 grams
Fiber: <1 gram
Fat: 5.89 grams
Saturated fat: 2.7 grams

1. Place a coffee filter in a fine-mesh sieve, set over a bowl, or line sieve with a double thickness of cheesecloth. Place yogurt in lined sieve. Cover and chill overnight.

2. Discard liquid in the bowl. Place yogurt in a food processor. Add cream cheese, avocado, green onions, garlic, cumin, lemon juice, hot pepper sauce, chili powder, and salt. Process for 1 minute or until smooth. Stir in cilantro.

3. Transfer to a serving bowl. Serve immediately with sliced jicama or zucchini or cover and chill for up to 1 week.

Tasty Tidbits

Use a natural brand of yogurt that doesn't contain gums, gelatin, or fillers. These ingredients may prevent the liquid whey from separating from the yogurt curd in step 1.

Ham, Pepper, and Mozzarella Pizza

The nutty flavor of stone-ground bread accents the fresh pizza ingredients.

Yields 4 pizzas
Prep time: 10 minutes
Cook time: 2–3 minutes
Serving size: 1 pizza
Each serving:
Glycemic index: low
Glycemic load: 9
Calories: 208
Protein: 22 grams
Carbohydrates: 17 grams
Fiber: 2 grams
Fat: 5.75 grams
Saturated fat: 1.42 grams

4 thin slices stone-ground bread

1 red bell pepper

1 yellow bell pepper

8 ounces sliced lean, 5 percent fat ham

3 TB. chopped black olives

3 oz. part skim milk mozzarella cheese, sliced

Freshly ground black pepper

1. Lightly toast stone-ground bread on both sides until golden.

2. Cut peppers into thick strips and arrange on toasted bread with ham. Sprinkle with black olives. Arrange mozzarella slices on top.

3. Grind pepper over all slices. Place under a hot broiler for 2–3 minutes until cheese is bubbling.

Spicy Chicken Lettuce Wraps

The chicken is highlighted with an Asian flavor.

Yields 8 wraps
Prep time: 30 minutes, plus 1 hour chill time
Cook time: 5 minutes
Serving size: 1 wrap
Each serving:
Glycemic index: very low
Glycemic load: 0
Calories: 50
Protein: 8 grams
Carbohydrates: 2 grams
Fiber: 2 grams
Fat: 1.5 grams
Saturated fat: <1 gram

8 oz. uncooked ground chicken or turkey breast

¼ cup chopped onion

1¼ cups shredded broccoli (broccoli slaw)

2 green onions, thinly sliced

2 TB. soy sauce or fish sauce

¼ cup chopped fresh cilantro

¼ tsp. crushed red pepper flakes

¼ tsp. salt

8 large butter lettuce leaves

1. In a medium nonstick skillet over medium heat, cook chicken or turkey and onion for 5 minutes or until chicken is brown and onion is tender. Drain mixture.

2. In a large bowl, combine chicken mixture, broccoli, green onions, soy sauce, cilantro, crushed red pepper, and salt. Cover and chill for 1 to 24 hours.

3. Divide mixture evenly among 8 lettuce leaves. Bring all sides of each lettuce leaf up to the center to form a bundle. Serve.

Blue Cheese Burgers

You'll forego the bun with these burgers, but not the meaty flavor coupled with blue cheese.

1 lb. extra-lean ground beef	**1 tsp. prepared Dijon mustard**
¼ cup finely chopped onion	**¼ cup crumbled blue cheese**
1 celery stalk, chopped	**4 lettuce leaves**
Salt and freshly ground black pepper	**1 tomato, sliced**
1 tsp. dried oregano	**4 dill pickle slices**

1. Preheat the broiler to high.

2. Place ground beef in a bowl with chopped onion and celery. Mix together, and season with salt and pepper.

3. Stir in oregano and Dijon mustard, and bring together to form a firm mixture.

4. Divide mixture into 8 equal portions. Place 4 on a cutting board and flatten each one slightly.

5. Place crumbled cheese in the center of each burger.

6. Flatten remaining mixture portions and place on top. Mold mixture together, enclosing crumbled cheese, and shape into 4 burgers.

7. Broil for 10 minutes or until cooked, turning once. Serve on a lettuce leaf with tomato slices and dill pickle.

Yields 4 burgers
Prep time: 15 minutes
Cook time: 10 minutes
Serving size: 1 burger
Each serving:
Glycemic index: very low
Glycemic load: 0
Calories: 242
Protein: 34 grams
Carbohydrates: 4 grams
Fiber: 1 gram
Fat: 10 grams
Saturated fat: 5 grams

Home-Cooked Goodness

Make burgers—hold the bun—your family tradition. Replace the bun with a freshly tossed green salad, red and green pepper rings, or baked sweet potato sticks.

Pickled Eggs

The eggs offer high-quality protein with a tangy taste treat.

1 cup vinegar	**1 TB. salt**
1 cup water	**1 TB. sugar**
1 TB. pickling spice	**12 hard-boiled eggs, shelled**

1. In a saucepan over medium heat, heat vinegar, water, pickling spice, salt, and sugar. Cook for 5 minutes.

2. Place hard-boiled eggs in a glass-lidded container, and pour hot vinegar mixture over top. Refrigerate for 3 days before serving. Eggs will keep 6 months in refrigerator.

Home-Cooked Goodness

Pickled eggs are great to have on hand. Cut in half and arrange on an appetizer platter with cheeses, sliced meats, and pickles. Or enjoy with an apple for a quick lunch or breakfast.

Yields 12 eggs

Prep time: 15 minutes
Cook time: 5 minutes
Serving size: 1 egg

Each serving:
Glycemic index: very low
Glycemic load: <1
Calories: 73
Protein: 7 grams
Carbohydrates: <1 gram
Fiber: 0 grams
Fat: 5 grams
Saturated fat: 1.6 grams

Sun-Dried Tomato Cheese Spread

Enjoy the taste of the Mediterranean sunshine with this quick and easy spread.

1 (8-oz.) package low-fat cream cheese at room temperature	**1 small clove garlic, minced (optional)**
2 TB. chopped sun-dried tomatoes (not oil packed)	**¼ tsp. salt**
1 tsp. dried chives	**Fresh vegetables cut for dipping, such as carrots, broccoli, sugar-snap peas, jicama, and cucumber spears**

In a small bowl, combine cream cheese, dried tomatoes, chives, garlic (if using), and salt. Stir to combine. Spoon spread on fresh vegetables.

Yields 1 cup spread

Prep time: 5 minutes, plus 24 hours chill time
Serving size: 2 tablespoons spread

Each serving:
Glycemic index: very low
Glycemic load: <1
Calories: 67
Protein: 3 grams
Carbohydrates: 3 grams
Fiber: 0 grams
Fat: 5 grams
Saturated fat: 3 grams

Ham and Cheddar Vegetable Snacks

The classic blending of ham and cheese gives a savory sweet and tangy flavor for vegetables.

1 (8-oz.) package low-fat cream cheese with chive and onions at room temperature

½ tsp. Dijon mustard

1 TB. mayonnaise

⅓ cup finely chopped, lean 5 percent fat ham

¼ cup shredded Cheddar cheese

Cut raw vegetables: celery sticks, cucumber, carrot sticks, jicama, radishes

1. In a small mixing bowl, stir together cream cheese, mustard, and mayonnaise. Stir in ham and Cheddar cheese.

2. Spread on raw vegetables. Can be stored in the refrigerator for up to 5 days.

Yields 1½ cups spread
Prep time: 10 minutes
Cook time: none
Serving size: ¼ cup spread
Each serving:
Glycemic index: very low
Glycemic load: 0
Calories: 120
Protein: 5 grams
Carbohydrates: 1 gram
Fiber: 0 grams
Fat: 10.7 grams
Saturated fat: 5.65 grams

Ham and Olive Pita Bread Sandwich

The sweet flavor of the ham combines well with a tangy olive tapenade.

1 TB. mayonnaise	**2 oz. sliced provolone cheese**
1 whole-wheat pita bread, sliced in half	**2 TB. olive tapenade**
4 oz. sliced deli baked lean 5 percent ham	

1. Spread mayonnaise on inside of pita bread.

2. Divide ham and cheese and place inside each half of pita bread.

3. Spread 1 tablespoon olive tapenade in each half.

4. Place both halves on microwave dish. Microwave on high for 30–45 seconds until cheese melts slightly.

5. Serve while warm.

Variation: Substitute turkey or salami for the ham.

Yields 1 sandwich
Prep time: 10 minutes
Cook time: 30–45 seconds in microwave
Serving size: ½ sandwich
Each serving:
Glycemic index: low
Glycemic load: 8
Calories: 305
Protein: 23 grams
Carbohydrates: 15 grams
Fiber: 2 grams
Fat: 17 grams
Saturated fat: 6.1 grams

Tasty Tidbits

This sandwich is also known as a *muffaletto* in Southern regional cuisine.

Chapter **8**

Appetizers and Hors d'Oeuvres

In This Chapter

- ♦ Appetite pleasers before the main course
- ♦ Flavors to suit many entrées
- ♦ Several starters can make a meal

The recipes in this chapter give you lots of variety and many choices. Serve appetizers before dinner, or cook several different ones to serve as a tapas dinner. Make double or triple servings of appetizers and call them lunch or brunch.

We included six variations on deviled eggs—a favorite low-glycemic package of high-quality protein, some fat, seasonings, and perhaps a vegetable garnish.

Each recipe contains farm-sourced ingredients, and not factory-sourced ones with mystery ingredients. This keeps the flavors and tastes clear while making the recipes more appealing and satisfying.

Grilled Salmon Tacos

Yields 32 tacos
Prep time: 1 hour
Cook time: 8 minutes on grill
Serving size: 1 small taco
Each serving:
Glycemic index: low
Glycemic load: 6
Calories: 119
Protein: 8 grams
Carbohydrates: 14 grams
Fiber: 3 grams
Fat: 3.4 grams
Saturated fat: 1.22 grams

This grilled salmon is tantalizingly flavored with hot and zingy chipotle chile and Southwestern toppings: sour cream and salsa.

2 lbs. fresh or frozen skinless salmon fillets

1 TB. ground chipotle chile pepper

¾ tsp. salt

2 cups green salsa

⅓ cup lime juice, bottled or fresh

¾ tsp. salt

1 (15-oz.) can black beans, drained

12 green onions, thinly sliced

1 cup chopped fresh cilantro

32 (4-inch) corn tortillas

1 (8-oz.) pkg. sour cream

Lime wedges

1. Thaw fish, if frozen. Rinse. Pat dry.

2. In a small bowl, combine chipotle chile pepper and ³/₄ teaspoon salt. Rub onto both sides of fish.

3. Place fish on greased grill rack directly over medium coals. Grill, uncovered, for 4 to 6 minutes per ¹/₂-inch thickness or until fish flakes easily when tested with a fork. Cool slightly. Break salmon into chunks.

4. In a large bowl, stir together salsa, lime juice, and ³/₄ teaspoon salt. Add salmon, black beans, green onions, and cilantro. Stir gently.

5. Divide salmon mixture among tortillas. Top each with a dollop of dairy sour cream. Serve with lime wedges.

Hummus and Artichoke Spread

Traditional Middle Eastern flavors of hummus, tomatoes, and feta cheese compliment marinated artichokes.

1 (7-oz.) pkg. hummus

¼ tsp. crushed red pepper flakes

½ cup sun-dried tomato pesto

1 (12-oz.) jar marinated artichokes, drained and coarsely chopped

4 oz. basil-and-tomato-flavored feta cheese

2 TB. minced green onion

1. Preheat the oven to 475°F.

2. Spread hummus on an ovenproof serving dish. Sprinkle with crushed red pepper. Top with spoonfuls of pesto and artichokes. Sprinkle with cheese and green onion.

3. Bake for 6 to 8 minutes or until cheese is softened. Serve with cut-up vegetables or stone-ground crackers.

Yields 3 cups dip
Prep time: 15 minutes
Cook time: 6 to 8 minutes
Serving size: ½ cup dip
Each serving:
Glycemic index: low
Glycemic load: 4
Calories: 225
Protein: 12 grams
Carbohydrates: 15 grams
Fiber: 7 grams
Fat: 13 grams
Saturated fat: 3 grams

Olive Tapenade Relish

Enjoy this tangy tapenade as an appetizer spread and as a topping for meats and seafood.

¾ cup whole pimiento-stuffed green olives, coarsely chopped

½ cup chopped black olives

⅓ cup chopped onion

¼ cup snipped fresh cilantro

2 TB. capers, drained

1 small fresh chile pepper, seeded and chopped

½ tsp. minced garlic

4 TB. finely chopped almonds

1 TB. white-wine vinegar

⅛ tsp freshly ground black pepper

1. In a bowl, combine green and black olives, onion, cilantro, capers, chile pepper, garlic, almonds, vinegar, and black pepper.

2. Serve on rye crispbread, deviled eggs, cut raw vegetables, or steamed and buttered vegetables. Or serve on cooked fish or pork.

Yields 1½ cups relish
Prep time: 15 minutes
Cook time: None
Serving size: ¼ cup relish
Each serving:
Glycemic index: very low
Glycemic load: <1
Calories: 92
Protein: 1 gram
Carbohydrates: 1 gram
Fiber: 2 grams
Fat: 9.3 grams
Saturated fat: 1.13 grams

Cheese Chips with Bean Dip

Your favorite corn chips become flavored with chile and cheese and hold the cilantro-flavored bean dip.

1 (16-oz.) can refried beans (no added fats)	¼ ground black pepper
1 TB. fresh lime juice	2 tsp. freshly chopped cilantro for garnish
½ red chile, seeded and finely chopped	1 (5-oz.) bag corn tortilla chips
3 tomatoes, finely chopped	2 TB. grated aged cheddar cheese
2 TB. chopped fresh cilantro	
¼ tsp. salt	¼ tsp. chili powder

1. Place refried beans in a mixing bowl. Mash lightly with fork against side of the bowl.

2. Add lime juice, red chile, tomatoes, cilantro, salt, and pepper, and stir to blend ingredients.

3. To make chips, preheat the broiler on low. Place corn chips on baking sheet. Mix grated cheese with chili powder, sprinkle over chips, and broil for 1–2 minutes, until cheese melts.

4. Serve bean dip in a bowl surrounded by chips. Garnish dip with cilantro.

Variation: Substitute 2 avocados for the bean dip to make guacamole.

Home-Cooked Goodness

Beans are high in fiber and protein; they make an taste-satisfying low-glycemic dip.

Yields 4 cups dip

Prep time: 15 minutes

Cook time: 2–3 minutes

Serving size: ½ cup dip and 6 chips

Each serving:

Glycemic index: low

Glycemic load: 6

Calories: 133

Protein: 4 grams

Carbohydrates: 13 grams

Fiber: 2 grams

Fat: 5.5 grams

Saturated fat: 1.18 grams

Deviled Eggs with 6 Variations

Dress up deviled eggs with a variety of flavors.

12 hard-boiled eggs, peeled

1. Slice eggs in half and carefully remove yolks. Place in a mixing bowl.

2. Prepare one or more of the fillings suggested in the variations that follow.

3. Fill eggs. Refrigerate until serving.

Variation 1: Classic Deviled Eggs

Enjoy preparing this classic version seasoned with mustard and parsley.

Gently moisten egg yolks with just enough mayonnaise so they hold together. Add …

1 tsp. dry mustard	**½ tsp. salt**
1 TB. finely chopped parsley	

Repack eggs with mixture and sprinkle with paprika, or if you like a hotter taste, a small amount of cayenne.

Variation 2: Bacon Deviled Eggs

Basil and bacon filling is topped with a cherry tomato.

Gently moisten egg yolks with just enough mayonnaise so they hold together. Add …

3 TB. chopped crisp bacon	**½ tsp. salt**
1 TB. chopped basil	**6 small cherry tomatoes, cut in half**

Repack eggs with mixture, and top with ½ small cherry tomato.

Variation 3: Smoked Salmon Deviled Eggs

An elegant egg with sour cream, smoked salmon, and chives.

Yields 24 filled eggs

Prep time: 15 minutes

Cook time: none

Serving size: 1 egg—2 halves

Each serving:

Glycemic index: very low to low, based on choice of variation

Glycemic load: <1

Calories: 78

Protein: 8 grams

Carbohydrates: <1 gram

Fiber: 0 grams

Fat: 5 grams

Saturated fat: 1.6 grams

Gently moisten egg yolks with just enough mayonnaise so they hold together. Stir in …

3 TB. finely chopped smoked salmon	**1 TB. caviar or smoked salmon**
1 TB. finely chopped chives	**Sprinkle paprika**

Repack eggs with mixture, and top with either a small dab of caviar or a sliver of smoked salmon and a sprinkle of paprika.

Variation 4: Tuna Deviled Eggs

Tuna is accented with pickle relish, pecans, and capers.

Gently moisten egg yolks with just enough mayonnaise so they hold together. Stir in …

3 TB. flaked tuna	**2 TB. finely chopped pecans**
2 TB. sweet pickle relish	**3 capers**

Repack egg whites with mixture, and top each with 3 capers.

Variation 5: Fruited Deviled Eggs

The sweetness of apples and raisins is accented with Parmesan.

Gently moisten egg yolks with just enough mayonnaise so they hold together. Stir in …

2 TB. grated Parmesan cheese	**2 TB. finely chopped apples**
	1 TB. finely chopped raisins

Repack egg whites with mixture and top with a small piece of shaved Parmesan cheese.

Variation 6: Avocado Deviled Eggs

Each egg holds the hot and spicy chile taste.

Gently moisten egg yolks with …

3 TB. mashed avocado and just enough mayonnaise so they hold together. Stir in …	**A pinch of cumin**
	⅛ tsp. garlic salt
3 TB. finely chopped tomato	**Coarsely grated fresh black pepper**
¼ tsp. chili powder	

Repack egg whites with mixture and coarsely grated fresh black pepper on each egg.

Mushroom Squares

Intense mushroom flavor accented with sweet nutmeg and spicy cayenne.

4 TB. olive oil

2 cups chopped mushrooms

½ cup finely chopped onions

4 eggs, lightly beaten

1 cup low-fat milk

1 cup yogurt, plain, low-fat

¼ tsp. nutmeg

⅛ tsp. cayenne

½ tsp. salt

⅛ tsp. freshly ground black pepper

Yields 1 (9-inch) crustless pie
Prep time: 20 minutes
Cook time: 25 minutes
Serving size: ⅛ pie
Each serving:
Glycemic index: very low
Glycemic load: 1
Calories: 147
Protein: 8 grams
Carbohydrates: 5 grams
Fiber: 1 gram
Fat: 10.5 grams
Saturated fat: 2.43 grams

1. Preheat the oven to 450°F.

2. In a skillet, heat 2 tablespoons olive oil over medium heat. Sauté mushrooms until wilted. Cover and cook over low heat 10 minutes.

3. Add 2 tablespoons olive oil and onions, and cook until onions are wilted.

4. In mixing bowl, combine eggs, milk, yogurt, nutmeg cayenne, salt, and pepper. Stir in mushrooms and onion. Pour into a lightly oiled 9-inch pie pan.

5. Bake 15 minutes, then reduce oven temperature to 350 degrees. Bake about 10 minutes longer until a knife inserted into pie comes out clean.

6. Cut into bite-size pieces and serve warm.

Home-Cooked Goodness

You can also prepare Mushroom Squares as a crustless quiche for lunch or brunch.

Mediterranean Chicken Quesadillas

Crisp, pan-fried quesadillas hold oregano-flavored shrimp, hummus, and artichoke hearts topped with feta cheese.

Yields 4 (8-inch) quesadillas
Prep time: 20 minutes
Cook time: 4 to 6 minutes per tortilla
Serving size: ¹/₂ quesadilla
Each serving:
Glycemic index: low
Glycemic load: 8
Calories: 236
Protein: 14
Carbohydrates: 18 grams
Fiber: 7 grams
Fat: 12 grams
Saturated fat: 3.36 grams

4 (8-inch) whole-wheat tortillas, preferably low-carb

¹/₃ cup plain or flavored hummus

1 cup shredded cooked lean chicken breast

1 (6.5-oz.) jar marinated artichoke hearts, drained and coarsely chopped

1 (4-oz.) pkg. crumbled low-fat feta cheese

1 tsp. oregano

4 TB. olive oil

1. Place tortillas on a work surface. Spread with hummus. Top half of each tortilla with shredded chicken, artichokes, cheese, and ¹/₄ teaspoon oregano. Fold tortillas in half, pressing gently.

2. Heat oil in a large skillet over medium heat for 1 minute. Cook quesadillas, 2 at a time, for 4–6 minutes or until browned and heated through, turning once. Cut each in half and serve.

 Glycemic Notes _____

If you prefer to keep the glycemic index value of the quesadillas lower, skip the whole-wheat tortillas. Instead, place ingredients in layers on an over-proof serving dish. Place under low broiler until cheese is barely melted. Serve on lettuce leaves. Eat with a fork.

Sun-Dried Tomato Spread

Enjoy this tangy yet sweet dip with cut raw vegetables.

12 medium sun-dried tomatoes (not packed in oil)

1 to 2 cups boiling water to cover sun-dried tomatoes

1 (8-oz.) package low-fat cream cheese, softened

½ cup chopped black olives (preferably kalamata)

¼ cup chopped pimento-stuffed green olives

¼ cup chopped red onion

Salt and pepper

Yields 2 cups spread
Prep time: 15 minutes, plus 1 hour chill time
Cook time: none
Serving size: ¼ cup spread
Each serving:
Glycemic index: low
Glycemic load: 2
Calories: 67
Protein: 2 grams
Carbohydrates: 8 grams
Fiber: 1 gram
Fat: 9 grams
Saturated fat: 3.12 grams

1. Place sun-dried tomatoes in a small bowl. Pour enough boiling water over tomatoes to cover. Let tomatoes stand until soft—about 10 minutes. Pat tomatoes dry and chop finely.

2. Mix cream cheese in a medium bowl until smooth. Mix in black olives, green olives, onion, and sun-dried tomatoes. Season to taste with salt and pepper.

3. Cover and refrigerate 1 hour or more. Let stand at room temperature for 1 hour before serving.

Mozzarella, Basil, and Tomato Tapas

Basil lends a peppery freshness to tomatoes and mozzarella.

2 TB. olive oil

1 tsp. minced garlic

1 loaf sourdough bread, cut into ⅜-inch slices, halved

1½ lbs. fresh mozzarella sliced to fit on top of bread slices

6 vine-ripened tomatoes, sliced

1 package fresh basil leaves

Yields 20 tapas
Prep time: 15 minutes
Cook time: 2 minutes
Serving size: 1 tapas
Each serving:
Glycemic index: low
Glycemic load: 9
Calories: 186
Protein: 12 grams
Carbohydrates: 16.5 grams
Fiber: 1 gram
Fat: 8 grams
Saturated fat: 4 grams

1. Preheat broiler on low broil.

2. Combine olive oil and garlic, and brush on top of bread slices.

3. Place fresh mozzarella slices on top bread. Place tomato slices on top cheese, and one basil leaf on top tomato.

4. Place under the broiler until cheese begins to melt. Serve hot.

Teriyaki Beef Skewers

Tender beef acquires an exciting flavor with tangy salty soy sauce and hot ginger.

Yields 12 appetizers
Prep time: 15 minutes
Cook time: 2 minutes
Serving size: 2 skewers
Each serving:
Glycemic index: very low
Glycemic load: 0
Calories: 248
Protein: 37 grams
Carbohydrates: 1 gram
Fiber: 0 grams
Fat: 10.7 grams
Saturated fat: 3.6 grams

½ cup soy sauce

2 TB. dry sherry

1 TB. finely chopped fresh ginger root

1 tsp. honey

2 green onions, chopped

2 lbs. lean round steak with visible fat trimmed, cut into strips, ¼ inch thick and 1½ inches long

12 bamboo skewers

1. Soak bamboo skewers in water.

2. In a large bowl, combine soy sauce, sherry, ginger root, honey, and green onions. Add meat and marinate 30 minutes.

3. Preheat the grill to high.

4. Thread meat pieces on the bamboo skewers. Grill for 3 minutes. Serve.

Pecan Brie

Warm creamy cheese is sweetened with brown sugar and pecans.

Yields 16 oz. cheese with ¾ cup pecans
Prep time: 15 minutes
Cook time: 2 minutes
Serving size: 1 oz. cheese and 2½ tsp. pecans
Each serving:
Glycemic index: low
Glycemic load: 3
Calories: 176
Protein: 7 grams
Carbohydrates: 4 grams
Fiber: 1 gram
Fat: 14 grams
Saturated fat: 5 grams

3 TB. packed brown sugar

¼ cup strong, freshly brewed coffee

¾ cup pecan halves

1 (16-oz.) round Brie cheese

1. In a medium skillet over medium heat, combine brown sugar and coffee. Stir until sugar is dissolved. Add pecans. Simmer until hot. Remove from heat.

2. Place Brie on a microwave-safe serving plate. Spoon pecan mixture on top.

3. Microwave on high for 1–2 minutes until cheese softens.

4. Serve on fresh fruit slices or stone-ground crackers.

Variation: Substitute coffee liquor for the coffee.

Chapter 9

Sauces and Condiments

In This Chapter

- ◆ Adding special tastes to your meals
- ◆ Spicing up grilled meats and leftovers
- ◆ Savory and sweet flavors

Condiments, sauces, and dips can enliven the most "boring" foods and leftovers. Even a leftover hamburger can once again delight your taste buds when served with a tapenade, salsa, or cream cheese dip.

Among the recipes in this chapter, we offer you two recipes for low-glycemic barbeque sauce—one that's spicy and one that's tangy. You'll find a number of salsas, and both a mild and robust olive relish, or tapenade.

Citrus and Apricot Spread

Enjoy this tangy citrus-flavored spread at breakfast or for afternoon snacks.

Yields 1½ cups spread
Prep time: 15 minutes
Cook time: none
Serving size: ¼ cup spread
Each serving:
Glycemic index: low
Glycemic load: 5
Calories: 111
Protein: 3 grams
Carbohydrates: 10 grams
Fiber: 0 grams
Fat: 6.6 grams
Saturated fat: 4.2 grams

1 (8-oz.) pkg. low-fat cream cheese, softened

1 TB. fresh orange peel, finely shredded

1 TB. fresh orange juice

1 TB. fresh lemon peel, finely shredded

1 TB. fresh lemon juice

¼ cup unsweetened apricot preserves

Raw vegetables such as celery, jicama, radishes, carrots, broccoli, cauliflower, or pea pods

1. In a small bowl, beat cream cheese, orange peel, orange juice, lemon peel, and lemon juice with an electric mixer on medium speed for 5 minutes or until smooth. Stir in preserves.

2. Serve with cut-up raw vegetables, such as celery, jicama, radishes, carrots, broccoli, cauliflower, and pea pods. Also delicious with pork and beef.

Nectarine-Avocado Salsa

Jalapeño pepper heats up the flavor of nectarines and avocados.

Yields 2¼ cups salsa
Prep time: 20 minutes
Cook time: none
Serving size: ¼ cup salsa
Each serving:
Glycemic index: low
Glycemic load: 1
Calories: 40
Protein: <1 gram
Carbohydrates: 4 grams
Fiber: <1 gram
Fat: 2.4 grams
Saturated fat: .34 grams

2 medium nectarines, seeded and chopped

1 small avocado (5 oz.), seeded, peeled, and chopped

¼ cup red bell pepper, chopped

2 TB. red onion (¼ of small onion), chopped

½ fresh jalapeño pepper, seeded and finely chopped, to taste

1 tsp. minced garlic

2 tsp. lime juice

¼ tsp. salt

¼ tsp. ground cumin

In a medium bowl, mix together nectarines, avocado, red bell pepper, onion, jalapeno pepper, garlic, lime juice, salt, and cumin. Cover and chill for up to 2 hours.

Gingered Date Spread

Here's a ginger- and date-flavored cream cheese, accented with raisins and pecans, then spread on apple slices.

1 (8-oz.) pkg. low-fat cream cheese, softened

2 TB. crystallized ginger, finely chopped

½ cup dates, chopped

2 TB. raisins, chopped

2 TB. pecans, finely chopped

4 large apples, sliced just before serving

Yields 2 cups spread
Prep time: 15 minutes
Cook time: none
Serving size: ⅛ cup spread, plus ¼ apple
Each serving:
Glycemic index: low
Glycemic load: 6
Calories: 84
Protein: 1 gram
Carbohydrates: 11 grams
Fiber: 1 gram
Fat: 4 grams
Saturated fat: 1.7 grams

1. In a small bowl, beat cream cheese with an electric mixer on medium speed until smooth.

2. Stir in ginger, dates, raisins, and pecans. Serve at once, or cover and chill overnight. Let chilled spread stand at room temperature about 30 minutes before serving. Spread on apple slices.

Carrot Horseradish Dip

A creamy veggie horseradish flavored with soy sauce and onions.

½ cup low-fat sour cream

½ (8-oz.) pkg. low-fat cream cheese, softened

¼ cup mayonnaise

2 tsp. soy sauce

1½ tsp. prepared horseradish

¼ tsp. salt

¼ tsp. ground black pepper

1½ cups carrots, shredded

¼ cup green onions, chopped

Celery sticks

Yields 3 cups dip
Prep time: 15 minutes
Cook time: none
Serving size: 3 celery sticks with 2 TB. spread each
Each serving:
Glycemic index: low
Glycemic load: <1
Calories: 45
Protein: 1 gram
Carbohydrates: 1 gram
Fiber: <1 gram
Fat: 9 grams
Saturated fat: 2.8 grams

1. In a medium-size mixing bowl, combine sour cream, cream cheese, mayonnaise, soy sauce, horseradish, salt, and pepper. Stir in shredded carrot and green onion.

2. Cut celery sticks in 4-inch lengths. Stuff celery sticks with spread. Store remaining spread in refrigerator for up to 1 week.

Cranberry Fruit Relish

This cranberry sauce is flavored with cinnamon, cloves, and nutmeg.

Yields 6 cups relish
Prep time: 15 minutes
Cook time: 15 minutes
Serving size: ¼ cup relish
Each serving:
Glycemic index: low
Glycemic load: 4
Calories: 37
Protein: <1 gram
Carbohydrates: 9 grams
Fiber: 1 gram
Fat: 0 grams
Saturated fat: 0 grams

1 (12-oz.) bag fresh cranberries

1 cup water

½ cup honey

1 apple (Pippin, Granny Smith, or Golden Delicious), cored and cut into ½-inch pieces

1 pear (Comice, D'Anjou, or Bosc), cored and cut into ½-inch pieces

Zest and juice of 1 orange

¼ tsp. ground cinnamon

¼ tsp. ground cloves

¼ tsp. ground nutmeg

2 TB. orange liqueur (optional)

1. In a medium saucepan over high heat, bring cranberries, water, and honey to a boil. Lower heat to medium-low. Add apple, pear, orange zest, orange juice, and spices.

2. Simmer for 10 minutes until cranberries pop. Cool to room temperature. Refrigerate until ready to serve. Stir in orange liqueur (if using) just before serving. Can be prepared several days in advance.

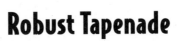

Robust Tapenade

A black olive spread flavored with anchovies, capers, and garlic.

Yields 1½ cups spread
Prep time: 10 minutes
Cook time: none
Serving size: 2 TB. spread
Each serving:
Glycemic index: very low
Glycemic load: 0
Calories: 67
Protein: <1 gram
Carbohydrates: 1 gram
Fiber: <1 gram
Fat: 7 grams
Saturated fat: .34 grams

¾ cup pitted black olives, such as Niçoise or Kalamata

6 anchovy fillets packed in olive oil, rinsed and patted dry

¼ cup capers, drained and rinsed

1 clove garlic, minced

⅓ cup olive oil

¼ tsp. freshly ground black pepper

1. In a food processor fitted with a chopping blade, combine olives, anchovies, capers, and garlic. With the motor running, drizzle in olive oil.

2. Continue to process, stopping to scrape down the sides of the bowl when necessary, until tapenade is puréed but still coarse. Transfer to a small bowl and season with pepper.

Olive Tapenade with Black Pepper

Here's a mild, black-olive spread flavored with bell peppers.

½ cup black olives, pitted and chopped

¼ cup red or green bell pepper, chopped

1 tsp. olive oil

1 tsp. red wine vinegar

1 tsp. coarsely ground black pepper

1. In a small bowl, stir together olives, peppers, olive oil, vinegar, and pepper. Tapenade will be chunky and not smooth.

2. Serve with meats, vegetables, as a sandwich spread, with eggs, or in omelets.

Variation: For a spread with more tang, substitute chopped green olives for the black olives.

Yields ¾ cup spread
Prep time: 10 minutes
Cook time: none
Serving size: 1 TB. spread
Each serving:
Glycemic index: very low
Glycemic load: 0
Calories: 31
Protein: 1 gram
Carbohydrates: 1 gram
Fiber: <1 gram
Fat: 3 grams
Saturated fat: <1 gram

Home-Cooked Goodness

Condiments like this add fabulous flavor to simply prepared foods. It's delicious on beef, pork, poultry, and lamb.

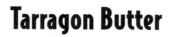

Tarragon Butter

This creamy butter spread is flavored with fresh tarragon and garlic.

¼ cup butter at room temperature

¼ cup olive oil

1 tsp. minced garlic

2 tsp. chopped fresh tarragon

In a mixing bowl, beat butter and olive oil with an electric mixer on medium speed for 30 seconds. Beat in garlic and tarragon.

Yields ½ cup spread
Prep time: 5 minutes
Cook time: none
Serving size: 1 TB.
Each serving:
Glycemic index: very low
Glycemic load: 0
Calories: 112
Protein: 0 grams
Carbohydrates: 0 grams
Fiber: 0 grams
Fat: 12.5 grams
Saturated fat: 4.58 grams

Tasty Tidbits

Tarragon butter adds an elegant touch to grilled meats, fish, and steamed vegetables.

Ginger Fruit Salsa

A sweet salsa flavored with mint and ginger.

Yields 2½ cups salsa
Prep time: 10 minutes
Cook time: none
Serving size: ⅓ cup salsa
Each serving:
Glycemic index: low
Glycemic load: 3
Calories: 32
Protein: <1 gram
Carbohydrates: 8 grams
Fiber: 1 gram
Fat: 0 grams
Saturated fat: 0 grams

1 mango, seeded, peeled, and chopped

1 cup fresh strawberries, chopped

½ cup fresh blueberries

1 TB. crystallized ginger, chopped

1 TB. fresh mint, chopped

Place mango, strawberries, blueberries, ginger, and mint in a small bowl and toss gently to combine.

Tasty Tidbits

Serve this sweet salsa as a side with salads, desserts, and seafood.

Coconut-Mango Salsa

A savory salsa exotically flavored with coconut and onion.

Yields 3 cups
Prep time: 30 minutes, plus 2 hours chill time
Cook time: none
Serving size: ¼ cup salsa
Each serving:
Glycemic index: low
Glycemic load: 2
Calories: 44
Protein: <1 gram
Carbohydrates: 6 grams
Fiber: 1 gram
Fat: 2.16 grams
Saturated fat: 1.91 grams

1 cup fresh coconut meat, chopped

2 medium ripe mangoes, peeled, seeded, and chopped

½ cup radishes, chopped

¼ cup green onions, sliced

1 TB. fresh ginger, grated

1 Serrano chile pepper, seeded and finely chopped

½ tsp. salt

1. In a food processor fitted with a chopping blade, purée coconut until smooth, adding a small amount of water if necessary.

2. In a mixing bowl, combine coconut purée, mangoes, radishes, onions, ginger, chile pepper, and salt. Stir to combine. Cover and chill for 2–6 hours.

Tasty Tidbits

The coconut adds an exotic flavor and will enhance the taste of grilled seafood and poultry.

Spicy Barbecue Sauce

A tomato-based sauce with a mild chile flavor.

1 cup onion (1 large), coarsely chopped

1 TB. olive oil

1 (14.5-oz.) can whole tomatoes with juice, chopped

1 (10.75-oz.) can tomato paste

⅔ cup cider vinegar

¼ cup orange juice

2 TB. Dijon-style mustard

2 TB. molasses

2 tsp. salt

1 tsp. chili powder

½ tsp. freshly ground black pepper

Yields 3½ cup sauce
Prep time: 20 minutes
Cook time: 30 minutes, plus 30 minutes cool time
Serving size: 3 TB. sauce
Each serving:
Glycemic index: low
Glycemic load: 3
Calories: 41
Protein: 1 gram
Carbohydrates: 7 grams
Fiber: 1 gram
Fat: <1 gram
Saturated fat: 0 grams

1. In a large saucepan over medium heat, sauté onion in olive oil about 8 minutes or until golden brown, stirring frequently. Stir in tomatoes, tomato paste, vinegar, orange juice, mustard, molasses, salt, chili powder, and pepper. Bring to a boil. Reduce heat. Simmer, uncovered, for 30–40 minutes, or until sauce is thickened, stirring occasionally. Remove from heat. Cool sauce for 30 minutes.

2. Transfer sauce, half at a time, to a blender or food processor. Cover and blend or process sauce until smooth. Refrigerate covered up to 1 month.

Tangy Barbecue Sauce

A tangy and sweet sauce flavored with hot peppers.

3 cups cider vinegar

2 TB. dark molasses or honey

1 TB. dry mustard

2–4 tsp. crushed red pepper

2 tsp. bottled hot pepper sauce

1½ tsp. salt

1½ tsp. ground black pepper

Yields 3¼ cups sauce
Prep time: 10 minutes, plus 6 hours stand time
Cook time: none
Serving size: 4 TB. sauce
Each serving:
Glycemic index: low
Glycemic load: 1
Calories: 12
Protein: 0 grams
Carbohydrates: 3 grams
Fiber: 0 grams
Fat: 0 grams
Saturated fat: 0 grams

In a clean 1-quart jar, mix together vinegar, molasses or honey, mustard, crushed red pepper, hot pepper sauce, salt, and black pepper. Cover and shake well. Let stand at room temperature for 6 hours to blend flavors. Refrigerate covered up to 7 days.

Poppy Seed Dressing

Vinaigrette flavored with tarragon and poppy seeds.

Yields 1½ cups dressing
Prep time: 10 minutes
Cook time: none
Serving size: 2 TB. dressing
Each serving:
Glycemic index: low
Glycemic load: 1
Calories: 170
Protein: 0 grams
Carbohydrates: 2 grams
Fiber: 0 grams
Fat: 18.6 grams
Saturated fat: 1.3 grams

1 tsp. dry mustard

1 tsp. paprika

¼ tsp. salt

1 tsp. dried tarragon

5 TB. vinegar

2 TB. honey

1 TB. lemon juice

2 TB. onion juice or finely grated onion

1 cup canola oil

1 TB. poppy seeds

1. Mix together mustard, paprika, salt, tarragon, and vinegar.

2. Add honey, lemon juice, and onion juice or onion. Gradually beat in oil. Chill.

3. Add poppy seeds just before serving on salads and fruit.

Cherry Vinaigrette

This savory vinaigrette is flavored with the fruit taste of cherries.

Yields ½ cup vinaigrette
Prep time: 5 minutes
Cook time: none
Serving size: 2 TB. vinaigrette
Each serving:
Glycemic index: low
Glycemic load: 6
Calories: 214
Protein: 0 grams
Carbohydrates: 13 grams
Fiber: 0 grams
Fat: 18.5 grams
Saturated fat: 1.3 grams

⅓ cup canola oil

¼ cup unsweetened cherry preserves

2 TB. cider vinegar

2 tsp. yellow mustard

In a jar with sealable lid, stir together oil, preserves, vinegar, and mustard. Cover tightly and shake. Store in the refrigerator.

Home-Cooked Goodness

The cherry taste will go well with tossed green salads, but don't stop there. Serve as a dressing for cold cuts, fruit, grilled meats, and holiday turkey.

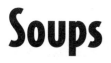

Chapter 10

Soups

In This Chapter

- Soups to match your entrée
- Main course soups
- Purées, vegetables, meats, and grains

The very word, soup, elicits feelings of comfort, being cared for, and easy evenings. Homemade soup is not as easy as opening a can and heating; however, we've designed these recipes so that many are almost as easy.

Chicken and Wild Rice Soup

This soup contains the exotic and crunchy taste of wild rice.

Yields 8 servings soup
Prep time: 20 minutes
Cook time: 25 minutes
Serving size: 1 cup soup
Each serving:
Glycemic index: low
Glycemic load: 3
Calories: 244
Protein: 23 grams
Carbohydrates: 10 grams
Fiber: 2 grams
Fat: 12.5 grams
Saturated fat: 3.6 grams

2 medium carrots, sliced
2 ribs celery, sliced
1 cup quartered mushrooms
3 TB. butter
3½ cups water
1 tsp. dried parsley
¾ tsp. ground black pepper

1 tsp. salt
1 tsp. thyme
⅛ tsp. ground cloves
½ tsp. paprika
4 (6-oz.) chicken breast halves, chopped
¾ cup cooked wild rice
1½ cups half-and-half

1. In a large saucepan, cook carrots, celery, and mushrooms in butter over medium heat until tender.

2. Add water, parsley, black pepper, salt, thyme, cloves, paprika, chicken, and wild rice. Cook and stir until mixture is bubbly and slightly thickened. Stir in half-and-half; heat through.

Onion Soup

A rich, beef-flavored onion broth topped with Parmesan cheese.

Yields 6 servings soup
Prep time: 10 minutes
Cook time: 40 minutes
Serving size: 1 cup soup
Each serving:
Glycemic index: very low
Glycemic load: 0
Calories: 77
Protein: 6 grams
Carbohydrates: 1 gram
Fiber: 0 grams
Fat: 5.4 grams
Saturated fat: 2.3 grams

1½ cups thinly sliced onions
4 cups cold water
1 TB. butter
1 TB. olive oil

6 cups natural beef broth
¼ tsp. freshly ground black pepper
6 TB. shredded Parmesan cheese (about ½ cup)

1. Soak sliced onions in cold water for 30 minutes. Drain.

2. In a large saucepan over medium heat, melt butter with olive oil and sauté onions until limp and lightly browned.

3. Add beef broth and pepper. Lower heat and simmer, covered for 30 minutes.

4. Spoon into serving bowls and top each with 1 tablespoon Parmesan.

Beef and Vegetable Stew

A mild stew flavored with sweet paprika and vegetables.

2 TB. olive oil

2 lbs. lean beef stew meat, cut into 1½-inch cubes

1 medium onion, sliced

2 tsp. minced garlic

1 tsp. salt

½ tsp. freshly ground black pepper

1 tsp. paprika

1 tsp. Worcestershire sauce

4 cups water

6 carrots, sliced

5 stalks celery, sliced

12 small red potatoes, cut in half

Yields 16 cups stew
Prep time: 20 minutes
Cook time: 2½ to 3½ hours
Serving size: 2 cups stew
Each serving:
Glycemic index: medium
Glycemic load: 16
Calories: 368
Protein: 33 grams
Carbohydrates: 29 grams
Fiber: 4 grams
Fat: 13.3 grams
Saturated fat: 4 grams

1. In a heavy skillet or Dutch oven, heat olive oil over medium heat, add meat, and cook until browned.

2. Add onion slices, garlic, salt, pepper, paprika, Worcestershire sauce, and water. Cover and simmer over low heat for 2–3 hours until meat is tender.

3. Add carrots, celery, and potatoes and simmer for 30 minutes until vegetables are tender.

Fresh Celery Soup with Parsley

An appealingly fresh-tasting soup to serve with lunch or as a snack.

1 bunch of celery ribs (entire stalk), finely sliced

2 cups water

2 TB. butter

3 TB. flour

½ tsp. dried parsley

¼ tsp. ground black pepper

½ tsp. salt

1 cup skim milk

Yields 4 cups soup
Prep time: 15 minutes
Cook time: 15 minutes
Serving size: ½ cup soup
Each serving:
Glycemic index: low
Glycemic load: 2
Calories: 59
Protein: 2 grams
Carbohydrates: 6 grams
Fiber: 2 grams
Fat: 3 grams
Saturated fat: 1.75 grams

1. In a saucepan, combine sliced celery and 2 cups water and bring to a boil. Cook until celery is tender.

2. In a saucepan, melt butter. Add flour, parsley, pepper, and salt. Cook, stirring for 2 minutes or until well blended. Add celery. Stir in skim milk. Heat until slightly thickened.

Mushroom Soup

Yields 6 servings soup
Prep time: 15 minutes
Cook time: 25 minutes
Serving size: 1¹/₂ cups soup
Each serving:
Glycemic index: low
Glycemic load: 2
Calories: 59
Protein: 3 grams
Carbohydrates: 5 grams
Fiber: 1 gram
Fat: 3 grams
Saturated fat: 1.66 grams

Intense mushroom flavor is accented with mild onion and black pepper.

1 TB. butter	½ tsp. salt
2 TB. chopped green onions	⅛ tsp. freshly ground black pepper
1 lb. mushrooms, sliced	
1 TB. flour	1½ cups nonfat half-and-half
4 cups natural chicken broth	

1. Melt butter in a saucepan over medium heat. Sauté green onion until tender. Add mushrooms and cook 5 minutes.

2. Sprinkle with flour and cook, while stirring, for 2 minutes.

3. Add chicken broth, salt, and pepper. Bring to a boil and simmer 5 minutes.

4. Add half-and-half and reheat without boiling. Serve.

Variation: Add ¹/₂ cup shredded cooked chicken to soup at step 3.

Barley Soup

Yields 6 servings soup
Prep time: 10 minutes
Cook time: 1 hour
Serving size: 1 bowl soup
Each serving:
Glycemic index: low
Glycemic load: 5
Calories: 144
Protein: 3 grams
Carbohydrates: 18 grams
Fiber: 7 grams
Fat: 6.7 grams
Saturated fat: 1.68 grams

A barley and vegetable soup finished with heavy cream and parsley.

1 cup pearl barley	3 ribs celery, cut in 1-inch pieces
1 onion, finely chopped	
1 TB. butter	1 tsp. salt
8 cups natural chicken broth	½ tsp. ground black pepper
2 carrots, cut in 1-inch slices	1 cup half-and-half (27 g fat)
	2 TB. chopped fresh parsley

1. Rinse barley in warm water and place in a soup pot.

2. Sauté onion in butter in a heavy skillet until tender.

3. In the soup pot, add the broth, carrot, celery, and onions. Add salt and pepper. Bring to a boil, cover and simmer about 1 hour until barley is tender.

4. Add half-and-half and parsley. Heat, and serve.

Tortilla Soup with Chicken

The spicy taste of this soup works as a starter or as a main course.

3 (6-inch) corn tortillas, cut into thin strips

2 TB. canola oil

1 cup purchased red or green salsa

3 cups water

2 cups cubed cooked chicken breast (12 oz.)

1 large zucchini, coarsely chopped

1 medium avocado, coarsely chopped

6 lime wedges (optional)

6 TB. sour cream

6 TB. chopped fresh cilantro

Yields 6 cups soup
Prep time: 20 minutes
Cook time: 25 minutes
Serving size: 1 cup soup
Each serving:
Glycemic index: low
Glycemic load: 8
Calories: 267
Protein: 18 grams
Carbohydrates: 24 grams
Fiber: 3 grams
Fat: 11 grams
Saturated fat: 2.95 grams

1. In a large skillet, sauté tortilla strips in oil until crisp; remove with a slotted spoon and drain on paper towels.

2. In a large saucepan, combine salsa, water, chicken, and zucchini. Simmer 20 minutes.

3. Serve in bowls. Divide avocado and tortilla among the bowls. Garnish with lime wedges (if using), 1 tablespoon sour cream, and 1 tablespoon cilantro.

After-the-Holiday Turkey Soup

Yields 14 cups soup
Prep time: 30 minutes
Cook time: 1³/₄ hours
Serving size: 2 cups soup
Each serving:
Glycemic index: low
Glycemic load: 5
Calories: 242
Protein: 28 grams
Carbohydrates: 16 grams
Fiber: 5 grams
Fat: 7.4 grams
Saturated fat: 2.5 grams

A good way to use leftover turkey—a delicious Italian-flavored soup.

1 meaty turkey frame, skin removed

4 cups water

1 large onion, quartered

2 cloves garlic, crushed

1 tsp. salt

3 cups carrots, sliced

¼ cup oil-packed sun-dried tomatoes, drained, cut into strips

2 tsp. dried Italian seasoning

1 TB. dried parsley

½ tsp. ground black pepper

1 (15-oz.) can black beans, rinsed and drained

1. Break turkey frame or cut in half with kitchen shears. Place in large stockpot. Add water, onion, garlic, and salt. Bring to boil. Simmer, covered, for 1½ hours.

2. Remove turkey frame. Cool. Cut meat off bones and chop coarsely. Set aside. Discard bones. Skim off fat.

3. Add carrots, sun-dried tomatoes, Italian seasoning, parsley, and pepper. Simmer, covered, for 10 minutes. Stir in turkey and beans; heat through.

Curried Chicken Vegetable Soup

A spicy chicken soup with vegetables, lentils, and golden raisins.

2 TB. olive oil

2 large chickens, about 12-oz. each, cut in pieces and skinned

1 onion, chopped

1 carrot, chopped

2 cups chopped celery

1 small turnip, chopped

1 TB. curry powder or to taste

4 whole cloves

6 black peppercorns, lightly crushed

¼ cup lentils

3¾ cups water

¼ cup golden raisins

Salt

Freshly ground black pepper

Yields 10 cups soup
Prep time: 20 minutes
Cook time: 1½ hours
Serving size: 1 cup soup
Each serving:
Glycemic index: low
Glycemic load: 3
Calories: 167
Protein: 18
Carbohydrates: 8 grams
Fiber: 2 grams
Fat: 7 grams
Saturated fat: 1.8 grams

1. Heat oil in a large saucepan and brown chicken. Transfer chicken to a plate.

2. Add onion, carrot, celery, and turnip to the saucepan and cook, stirring occasionally, until lightly softened. Stir in curry powder, cloves, and peppercorns. Cook for 1–2 minutes. Add lentils.

3. Pour water into the saucepan, bring to a boil, then add raisins, chicken, and any juices from the plate. Cover and simmer gently for about 1¼ hours.

4. Remove chicken from the pan and discard skin and bones. Chop chicken meat into bite-size chunks, return to the soup, and reheat. Season to taste with salt and pepper before serving.

Tasty Tidbits _____

This main-dish soup recipe originated in India and contains Indian cuisine spices like curry, cloves, and pepper. Turn up the heat of this dish by increasing the amounts of curry and freshly ground pepper you use.

Minestrone with Red Beans

Yields 16 cups soup
Prep time: 15 minutes
Cook time: 50 minutes
Serving size: 1 cup soup
Each serving:
Glycemic index: very low
Glycemic load: 2
Calories: 80
Protein: 9 grams
Carbohydrates: 8 grams
Fiber: 2 grams
Fat: 1.37 grams
Saturated fat: .58 grams

A meal in a bowl with plenty of vegetables and beans, and flavored with lean bacon.

2 TB. olive oil

2 tsp. minced garlic

1 onion, sliced

2 cups diced Canadian bacon, cooked, drained, and crumbled

2 small zucchini, quartered and sliced

1½ cups green beans, chopped

2 small carrots, diced

2 celery ribs, finely chopped

5 cups water

½ tsp. dried rosemary, crumbled

¼ tsp. salt

¼ tsp. ground black pepper

½ cup frozen peas

1 (7-oz.) can red kidney beans, dried and rinsed

1 cup shredded green cabbage

4 tomatoes, skinned and seeded

4 TB. grated Parmesan cheese

1. Heat oil in a large saucepan. Sauté garlic and onions for 5 minutes, until just softened. Add bacon, zucchini, green beans, carrots, and celery to the pan and sauté for another 3 minutes.

2. Pour 5 cups cold water over vegetables and add rosemary, salt, and pepper. Cover pan with a tight-fitting lid and simmer for 25 minutes.

3. Add peas and kidney beans and cook for 8 minutes. Add cabbage and tomatoes and cook for 5 minutes.

4. Serve soup in bowls. Sprinkle lightly with Parmesan cheese.

Roasted Acorn Squash Soup

A sophisticated autumn or winter soup that's thick and creamy.

2½ lbs. acorn squash

½ cup water

2 TB. olive oil

1½ cups diced onion (about 3 medium)

½ tsp. dried thyme, crushed

1 small bay leaf

1 tsp. cinnamon

½ tsp. salt

¼ tsp. freshly ground black pepper

3½ cups water

1 TB. honey

⅓ cup low-fat cream

½ tsp. freshly grated nutmeg

Yields 6 cups soup
Prep time: 10 minutes
Cook time: 40 minutes, plus bake 1 to 1½ hours
Serving size: 1 cup soup
Each serving:
Glycemic index: low
Glycemic load: 9
Calories: 168
Protein: 3 grams
Carbohydrates: 24 grams
Fiber: 3 grams
Fat: 4.9 grams
Saturated fat: 1.1 grams

1. Preheat the oven to 375°F.

2. Split squash in half lengthwise. With a spoon, scrape out seeds and fibers from cavity of squash. Place, flesh-side down, in a baking dish.

3. Add ½ cup water to baking pan. Bake 1 to 1½ hours until skin is brown and flesh is tender when pierced with a knife. Remove from the oven. When cool enough to handle, scoop out flesh and discard skin.

4. In a large saucepan, heat olive oil. Add onion, thyme, and bay leaf. Cook over medium heat, stirring often, until onion is tender and translucent, about 20 minutes.

5. Add squash, cinnamon, salt, and black pepper. Cook 5 minutes, stirring often.

6. Add water. Simmer, uncovered, for 20 minutes, stirring occasionally. Remove bay leaf. Stir in honey. Cool slightly. Purée soup, half at a time, in a blender or food processor.

7. Return soup to the pot and bring to simmer. Stir in cream and ¼ teaspoon grated nutmeg; heat through. Serve and sprinkle with remaining nutmeg.

Home-Cooked Goodness

By puréeing the soup, you obtain a creamy, thick soup that doesn't require thickening. This extra step gives you a luscious consistency and more flavor.

Hearty Vegetable Soup

Vegetables abound in this oregano-flavored soup.

Yields 10 cups soup
Prep time: 15 minutes
Cook time: 45 minutes
Serving size: about 1½ cups soup
Each serving:
Glycemic index: low
Glycemic load: 21
Calories: 235
Protein: 10 grams
Carbohydrates: 47 grams
Fiber: 9 grams
Fat: 1 gram
Saturated fat: 0 grams

6 cups water

1 (15-oz.) can pinto beans, drained

¼ cup dry lentils

¼ cup pearl barley

¼ cup chopped onion

½ cup sliced carrots

½ cup sliced celery

¼ cup chopped parsley

4 red potatoes, cut in quarters

1 TB. tomato paste

1 tsp. dried oregano

1 tsp. salt

½ tsp. freshly ground black pepper

½ cup frozen corn

½ cup frozen green beans

½ cup shredded fresh cabbage

1. In a large saucepan over high heat, bring water to a boil. Add pinto beans, lentils, barley, onion, carrots, celery, parsley, potatoes, tomato paste, oregano, salt, and pepper. Cover, reduce heat, and simmer for 30 minutes.

2. Add corn, green beans, and cabbage. Simmer, covered for 15 minutes.

Tasty Tidbits _____

Serve this soup for lunches or dinners with sliced meat or cheese for added protein.

Shrimp and Crab Chowder with Corn

A thick soup that's hearty and satisfying. Add a dinner salad as a side dish.

2 TB. olive oil	**1 cup peeled, cooked shrimp**
1 onion, chopped	**⅔ cup light cream**
1 (12-oz.) can corn, drained	**Pinch of cayenne**
1½ cups milk	**½ tsp. salt**
1 cup water	**¼ tsp. freshly ground black pepper**
1 (6-oz.) can white crabmeat, drained and flaked	

Yields 4 cups chowder
Prep time: 15 minutes
Cook time: 10 minutes
Serving size: 1 cup chowder
Each serving:
Glycemic index: low
Glycemic load: 7
Calories: 323
Protein: 29 grams
Carbohydrates: 18 grams
Fiber: 1 gram
Fat: 15 grams
Saturated fat: 10 grams

1. Heat olive oil in a large saucepan. Gently sauté onion for 4–5 minutes, until softened.

2. Add corn to saucepan, along with milk and water. Bring soup to a boil, then reduce heat, cover the pan with a tight-fitting lid, and simmer over low heat for 5 minutes.

3. Pour soup, in batches if necessary, into a blender or food processor. Process until smooth.

4. Return soup to the pan and stir in crabmeat, shrimp, cream, cayenne, salt, and pepper. Reheat gently over low heat.

Variation: For lower fat, substitute olive oil for the butter, use skim milk and low-fat cream (for calculation used nonfat half-and-half). Results: 242 calories, 6 grams fat, 3.5 grams saturated fat.

Sunny Gazpacho

The crisp, chilled cucumber, green bell peppers, and celery in a spicy tomato base add refreshing sparkle to summer lunches and dinners.

1 large cucumber	**1 tsp. dried basil**
1 large green bell pepper	**½ tsp. paprika**
3 ribs celery	**2 TB. olive oil**
1 green onion	**3 TB. fresh lemon juice**
¼ cup parsley	**4 cups fresh or low-sodium tomato juice**
½ tsp. freshly ground black pepper	

Yields 8 cups gazpacho

Prep time: 25 minutes, plus overnight chill time

Cook time: none

Serving size: 1 cup gazpacho

Each serving:

Glycemic index: low

Glycemic load: 2

Calories: 72

Protein: 2 grams

Carbohydrates: 7 grams

Fiber: 1 gram

Fat: 4 grams

Saturated fat: <1 gram

1. In food processor fitted with a chopping blade, finely chop cucumber and place in a large bowl. Repeat process of finely chopping green bell pepper, celery, green onion, and parsley, placing in the same large bowl after each process.

2. Stir in black pepper, basil, paprika, olive oil, and lemon juice. Stir in tomato juice.

3. Cover and chill overnight.

Tasty Tidbits

Select the freshest vegetables for this recipe. Use only fresh lemon juice or bottled fresh-squeezed organic lemon juice with no preservatives, available at health food groceries, if not in the health food section of your grocery store. This gives the soup a clear fresh taste.

Mediterranean Fish Stew

Shrimp, mussels, and white fish flavored with herbs and turmeric with a citrus note.

1 onion, chopped	1 bay leaf
1 carrot, diced	1 tsp. dried orange peel
3 tsp. minced garlic	½ tsp. salt
3 TB. olive oil	¼ tsp. freshly ground black pepper
½ tsp. ground turmeric	1 lb. white fish, skinned and chopped
⅔ cup dry white wine	2 cups cooked medium shrimp
1 (14-oz.) can chopped tomatoes	12 mussels or clams in shell
2 cups water	3 TB. fresh Parmesan cheese, shaved
1 TB. chopped fresh parsley	¼ cup chopped fresh parsley
1 tsp. dried thyme	
1 tsp. fennel seeds	

Yields 12 cups stew
Prep time: 20 minutes
Cook time: 40 minutes
Serving size: 2 cups stew
Each serving:
Glycemic index: low
Glycemic load: 2
Calories: 273
Protein: 33 grams
Carbohydrates: 8 grams
Fiber: 2 grams
Fat: 9.5 grams
Saturated fat: 1.6 grams

1. In a large saucepan over medium heat, sauté onion, carrot, and garlic in oil for about 6–7 minutes.

2. Stir in turmeric. Add wine, tomatoes, water, parsley, thyme, fennel seeds, bay leaf, orange peel, salt, and pepper. Bring to a boil, then cover. Reduce heat and simmer for 20 minutes.

3. Add fish and seafood to the pan and simmer for about 10 minutes, until mussels open. Remove bay leaf.

4. Garnish with Parmesan and fresh parsley.

Jerusalem Artichoke Soup

Enjoy this earthy and savory taste to warm your days and evenings.

Yields 6 cups soup	
Prep time: 15 minutes	
Cook time: 45 minutes	
Serving size: 1 cup soup	
Each serving:	
Glycemic index: low	
Glycemic load: 2	
Calories: 90	
Protein: 3 grams	
Carbohydrates: 6 grams	
Fiber: 1 gram	
Fat: 6 grams	
Saturated fat: 3.5 grams	

3 TB. butter

1 onion, chopped

1 lb. Jerusalem artichoke, peeled and cut into chunks

3¾ cups chicken stock

1 cup skim milk

⅛ tsp. saffron or turmeric

¼ tsp. salt

¼ tsp. ground black pepper

6 TB. chopped fresh parsley, to garnish

1. Melt butter in a large, heavy-based saucepan and cook onion for 5–8 minutes, until soft but not browned, stirring occasionally.

2. Add artichoke to the saucepan and stir until coated. Cover with a tight-fitting lid and cook gently for 10–15 minutes; do not allow artichoke to brown. Pour in stock and milk, then cover and simmer for 15 minutes. Cool slightly, then process in a food processor or blender until smooth.

3. Pour soup back into saucepan. Add saffron, salt, and pepper. Reheat gently. Serve with chopped parsley for garnish.

Part 4

Main Dishes

Choose from a wide variety of main course dishes based on meats, poultry, and seafood. If you have a yearning for a special type of food, chances are good you'll find a recipe for it here.

Main dish salads offer you a complete balanced meal. We've calculated the nutritional value of the salad dressings separately so you can choose exactly how much you want to eat based on your nutritional needs.

The vegetarian chapter gives you low-glycemic fare that's meat-free but contains plenty of protein and flavor.

Main Dish Salads

In This Chapter

- Adding high-quality protein to salads
- A perfect low-glycemic meal
- Using what's on hand

Main dish salads are the food of what's happening now. People want lighter fare, more vegetables, and healthier food. With a main dish salad, you're in control. You can manage the calorie count by choosing how much dressing you eat.

Not Your Ordinary Entrée

A main dish salad is the perfect low-glycemic meal. You'll eat at least two servings of vegetables/fruit, good fats, and lean high-quality protein. Packaged into this meal—sight unseen—are antioxidants, farm-sourced goodness, vitamins, fiber, and other health-boosting nutrients.

In these recipes, we give you nutritional counts for each salad and separately for each dressing. Additional nutritional counts for the dressings are per tablespoon so you can decide how much you want to eat based on your daily calorie and fat needs.

Chicken, Avocado, and Raspberry Salad

This elegant, mild-tasting salad is enhanced with the sweet tartness of fresh raspberries.

Yields 4 salads
Prep time: 15 minutes
Cook time: 15–20 min-utes
Serving size: 1 salad
Each serving:
Salad:
Glycemic index: low
Glycemic load: 5
Calories: 308
Protein: 30 grams
Carbohydrates: 10 grams
Fiber: 3 grams
Fat: 16.5 grams
Saturated fat: 2.95 grams
Salad dressing per TB.:
Glycemic index: low
Glycemic load: 0
Calories: 76
Carbohydrates: 2 grams
Fat: 8 grams
Saturated fat: 1 gram

1 TB. honey

1 TB. soy sauce

1 large chicken breast (about 1 lb.) skinned, boned, and halved

4 TB. olive oil

1 TB. red wine vinegar

1 TB. fruit jelly, any flavor

¼ tsp. salt

⅛ tsp. freshly ground black pepper

6 cups chopped fresh Bibb lettuce

2 avocados (6 oz. each), peeled, pitted, and cut into chunks

1 cup fresh raspberries

1. Preheat the oven to 425°F.

2. Blend honey and soy sauce together in a small bowl, then brush on chicken breast.

3. Place chicken in an oven-broiling pan. Roast for 15–20 minutes, until meat is cooked. Remove from the oven to cool.

3. To make dressing, put olive oil, vinegar, jelly, salt, and pepper in a small bowl and whisk.

4. Slice chicken breast diagonally and arrange on four individual plates with salad greens, avocados, and raspberries. Spoon desired amount of dressing on salads and serve.

Tasty Tidbits

Fresh berries always taste luxurious and a bit extravagant, while offering high amounts of healthful antioxidants.

Turkey and Ham Paella Salad

The spiced rice lends an exotic taste balanced with a touch of sweetness from raisins and bell peppers.

1 (8-oz.) pkg. basmati rice

3 cups chopped cooked turkey

1 cup chopped tomato

1 cup frozen sweet peas

1 cup chopped red bell pepper

⅓ cup golden raisins

¼ cup sliced green onion

½ cup cooked lean 5 percent ham, cut into thin strips

1 tsp. saffron or turmeric

4 TB. olive oil

2 TB. white wine vinegar

1 tsp. oregano

1 tsp. paprika

¼ tsp. salt

¼ tsp. freshly ground black pepper

⅓ cup sliced almonds, toasted

Yields 10 cups salad
Prep time: 25 minutes, plus 2 hours chill time
Cook time: 15 minutes
Serving size: 1⅔ cups salad
Each serving:
Salad:
Glycemic index: low
Glycemic load: 24
Calories: 327
Protein: 30 grams
Carbohydrates: 45 grams
Fiber: 6 grams
Fat: 3 grams
Saturated fat: <1 gram
Salad dressing per tablespoon:
Glycemic index: very low
Glycemic load: 0
Calories: 59
Carbohydrates: 0 grams
Fat: 6.5 grams
Saturated fat: <1 gram

1. Prepare rice according to package directions. Spread on a baking sheet, cover, and refrigerate about 20 minutes or until cool.

2. In a salad bowl, combine turkey, tomato, peas, bell pepper, raisins, green onion, and ham. Add rice and saffron or turmeric. Toss.

3. To make dressing, mix olive oil, vinegar, oregano, paprika, salt, and pepper in a small bowl. Add to salad and toss well.

4. Chill for 2 hours or longer. Serve with a slotted spoon or salad tongs. Sprinkle with almonds before serving.

Tuna Chutney Salad

A tuna salad that's sweet, tart, and salty with an Indian curry flavor.

Yields 8 cups salad
Prep time: 15 minutes
Cook time: none
Serving size: 1 cup salad
Each serving:
Salad:
Glycemic index: low
Glycemic load: 3
Calories: 183
Protein: 28 grams
Carbohydrates: 12 grams
Fiber: 2 grams
Fat: 2.5 grams
Saturated fat: <1 gram
Salad dressing per tablespoon:
Glycemic index: very low
Glycemic load: 0
Calories: 92
Carbohydrates: <1 gram
Fat: 10 grams
Saturated fat: 1.3 grams

2 cups diced cooked tuna

1 (13.25-oz.) can unsweetened pineapple tidbits, drained

1 cup sliced celery

¼ cup salted peanuts

¼ cup sliced green onions

1 cup chopped unpeeled apple

1 cup chopped cucumber

1 cup mayonnaise

3 TB. chopped chutney

½ tsp. grated fresh lime peel

2 TB. fresh lime juice

1 tsp. ground ginger

½ tsp. curry powder

¼ tsp. salt

8 lettuce leaves

1. Place tuna, pineapple, celery, peanuts, green onions, apple, and cucumber in a salad bowl.

2. To make dressing, combine mayonnaise, chutney, lime peel, lime juice, ginger, curry powder, and salt in a lidded jar and shake well.

3. Serve salad on lettuce leaves. Top with desired amount of dressing.

Home-Cooked Goodness

Stock canned tuna—either water-packed or oil-packed—in your pantry. You can substitute tuna in many main dish salads if you don't have the specific meat called for. Some canned tuna comes in solid chunks, and would work well in this salad.

Cobb Salad

A homemade vinaigrette blends with the blue cheese and avocado to give this salad a rich, savory, and creamy flavor.

6 cups torn Romaine lettuce

¼ pound turkey, sliced into strips

¼ pound lean 5 percent ham, sliced into strips

2 oz. Swiss cheese, sliced into strips

2 oz. cheddar cheese, sliced into strips

¼ cup black olives, sliced

2 tomatoes, chopped

1 avocado, sliced thick

2 TB. red wine vinegar

¼ cup olive oil

¼ tsp. salt

⅛ tsp. freshly ground black pepper

2 hard-cooked eggs, chopped

3 TB. crumbled blue cheese

1. Place lettuce on a large serving platter.

2. On top of lettuce, arrange turkey, ham, Swiss cheese, cheddar cheese, black olives, tomatoes, and avocado.

3. In a small jar with a tight-fitting lid, shake together vinegar, oil, salt, and pepper.

4. Top salad with eggs and blue cheese. Top with desired amount of dressing.

Yields 8 cups salad
Prep time: 20 minutes
Cook time: none
Serving size: 2 cups salad
Each serving:
Salad:
Glycemic index: very low
Glycemic load: 0
Calories: 369
Protein: 31 grams
Carbohydrates: 5 grams
Fiber: 3 grams
Fat: 25 grams
Saturated fat: 10 grams
Salad dressing per tablespoon:
Glycemic index: very low
Glycemic load: 0
Calories: 72
Carbohydrates: 0 grams
Fat: 8 grams
Saturated fat: <1 gram

Home-Cooked Goodness

Homemade blue cheese and vinaigrette dressing is the ultimate blue-cheese dressing. It's lower in fat than the commercial creamy type and gives you more of the blue cheese taste.

Tailgate Beef Salad

The rich taste of beef blends with savory black olives, mushrooms, and artichokes for tangy and satisfying flavor.

12 mushrooms, sliced	2 tsp. Dijon mustard
1–1½ lbs. cooked lean roast beef or flank steak, sliced into strips	1 tsp. minced garlic
	1 tsp. red chili powder
	1 tsp. salt
12 cherry tomatoes, halved	¼ tsp. freshly ground black pepper
½ cup pitted black olives	
1 green bell pepper, seeded and sliced into rings	1 head Romaine lettuce, sliced
1 (14-oz.) can artichoke hearts, drained and halved	2 TB. minced fresh parsley
	2 TB. crumbled blue cheese
1 TB. capers	4 slices salami, fried, blotted on paper towels, and crumbled
½ cup olive oil	
¼ cup red-wine vinegar	

Yields 12 cups salad

Prep time: 20 minutes, plus marinate overnight

Cook time: none

Serving size: 2 cups salad

Each serving:

Salad:

Glycemic index: very low

Glycemic load: 0

Calories: 269

Protein: 33 grams

Carbohydrates: 5 grams

Fiber: 3 grams

Fat: 13 grams

Saturated fat: 6.5 grams

Salad dressing per tablespoon:

Glycemic index: very low

Glycemic load: 0

Calories: 72

Carbohydrates: 0 grams

Fat: 8 grams

Saturated fat: 1 gram

1. In a food storage bowl or container, combine mushrooms, beef, tomatoes, black olives, green pepper, artichokes, and capers.

2. In a lidded jar, combine olive oil, red-wine vinegar, Dijon mustard, garlic, chili powder, salt, and pepper. Shake well.

3. To serve: Arrange beef mixture on bed of lettuce and parsley on individual plates or in a salad bowl. Sprinkle with bleu cheese and crumbled salami. Top with desired amount of dressing.

Crab Louis

Succulent cold crab on a bed of lettuce with creamy homemade Louis dressing has a slightly sweet and tangy flavor.

½ cup mayonnaise

1 tsp. Tomato paste

¼ cup olive oil

1 TB. lemon juice

2 TB. chili sauce

2 TB. minced fresh chives

2 TB. olives

½ tsp. horseradish

½ tsp. Worcestershire sauce

1 TB. sweet pickle relish

¼ tsp. salt

¼ tsp. ground black pepper

6 cups chilled lettuce, torn into bite-size pieces

3 cups cooked crabmeat, flaked

6 hard-boiled eggs, quartered

3 tomatoes, quartered

3 TB. capers

1. To make dressing, whisk mayonnaise, tomato paste, olive oil, lemon juice, chile sauce, chives, olives, horseradish, Worcestershire sauce, relish, salt, and pepper. Place in a jar with a tight-fitting lid. Chill.

2. Arrange lettuce in a shallow salad bowl and mound crabmeat on top. Spoon desired amount of dressing over crab and garnish with hard-cooked egg, tomatoes, and capers.

Home-Cooked Goodness

If you love this salad dressing, double the recipe and serve with raw or cooked vegetables, or as a sauce for grilled seafood.

Yields 12 cups crab salad

Prep time: 20 minutes

Cook time: none

Serving size: 2 cups crab salad

Each serving:

Salad:

Glycemic index: very low

Glycemic load: 0

Calories: 217

Protein: 38 grams

Carbohydrates: 5 grams

Fiber: 3 grams

Fat: 5 grams

Saturated fat: 2 grams

Salad dressing per tablespoon:

Glycemic index: very low

Glycemic load: 0

Calories: 74

Carbohydrates: <1 gram

Fat: 8 grams

Saturated fat: 1 gram

Niçoise Salad

Tarragon lends a peppery taste that sparkles with tangy capers and Dijon mustard.

Yields 15 cups salad	

Prep time: 20 minutes

Cook time: 10 minutes

Serving size: 2¹/₂ cups salad

Each serving:

Salad:

Glycemic index: low

Glycemic load: 12

Calories: 250

Protein: 17 grams

Carbohydrates: 32 grams

Fiber: 4 grams

Fat: 6 grams

Saturated fat: <1 gram

Salad dressing per tablespoon:

Glycemic index: very low

Glycemic load: 0

Calories: 81

Carbohydrates: 0 grams

Fat: 9 grams

Saturated fat: 1 gram

6 TB. olive oil

2 TB. tarragon vinegar

1 tsp. tarragon or Dijon mustard

1 tsp. minced garlic

¼ tsp. salt

⅛ tsp. freshly ground black pepper

1 cup green beans

12 small new potatoes

8 cups coarsely chopped Romaine lettuces

1 (7 oz.) can tuna packed in oil, drained

6 anchovy fillets, halved lengthwise and drained

12 pitted black olives

4 tomatoes, chopped

2 tsp. capers

2 hard-boiled eggs, chopped

1. Mix oil, vinegar, tarragon or mustard, garlic, salt, and pepper in a jar with tight-fitting lid. Shake to blend.

2. Cook green beans and potatoes in separate saucepans of boiling salted water until just tender. Drain and add to the bowl with lettuce, tuna, anchovies, olives, tomatoes, and capers. Toss with desired amount of dressing.

3. Just before serving, add eggs and toss well.

Tasty Tidbits _____

Flavored vinegars can change the flavor of a salad. Try several, such as balsamic, tarragon, red or white wine, or raspberry.

Ham and Garbanzo Bean Salad

A sparkling vinaigrette dressing imparts a rich, tangy flavor to the ham and beans.

1 (15-oz.) can garbanzo beans, drained and rinsed	2 TB. white wine vinegar
½ cup coarsely chopped lean 5 percent ham	¼ cup olive oil
	½ tsp. salt
¼ cup chopped green onions	¼ tsp. freshly ground black pepper
1 ripe tomato, cut into bite-size wedges	6 cups chopped Romaine lettuce
1 red bell pepper, seeded and cut into ½-inch pieces	3 TB. flax seeds
¼ cup finely chopped parsley	2 TB. shredded Parmesan cheese
1 tsp. minced garlic	

1. Place garbanzo beans, ham, green onions, tomato, red bell pepper, and parsley into a salad bowl.

2. In a jar with a tight-fitting lid, place minced garlic, vinegar, olive oil, salt, and pepper. Close the lid and shake to blend salad dressing.

3. Place lettuce in a large salad bowl. With a slotted spoon or salad tongs, spoon garbanzo bean mixture on lettuce. Add desired amount of dressing and toss. Sprinkle with flax seeds and Parmesan cheese.

Yields 6 servings salad

Prep time: 15 minutes
Cook time: none
Serving size: ⅙ salad

Each serving:
Salad:
Glycemic index: low
Glycemic load: 3
Calories: 73
Protein: 12 grams
Carbohydrates: 14 grams
Fiber: 6 grams
Fat: 1 gram
Saturated fat: <1 gram
Salad dressing per tablespoon:
Glycemic index: very low
Glycemic load: 0
Calories: 94
Carbohydrates: 0 gram
Fat: 10 grams
Saturated fat: 1 grams

Home-Cooked Goodness

You can sprinkle whole or ground flax seeds on any salad or vegetable. They look festive, and your body utilizes their omega-3 essential fatty-acid goodness whether whole or ground.

Sautéed Salmon Salad

Yields 1 lb. salmon with 5 cups vegetables

Prep time: 15 minutes

Cook time: 15 minutes

Serving size: ¼ lb. salmon and 1¼ cups vegetables

Each serving:

Salad:

Glycemic index: low

Glycemic load: 1

Calories: 223

Protein: 30 grams

Carbohydrates: 10 grams

Fiber: 2 grams

Fat: 7 grams

Saturated fat: <1 gram

Salad dressing per tablespoon:

Glycemic index: low

Glycemic load: 0

Calories: 76

Carbohydrates: 1 gram

Fat: 8 grams

Saturated fat: <1 gram

Asian-style sesame oil adds a warm flavor to this salad that's served warm.

2 TB. sesame oil

Grated rind of ½ orange

Juice of 1 orange

1 tsp. Dijon mustard

1 tsp. dried tarragon

Salt and freshly ground black pepper

1 lb. salmon (wild, lean) fillet, skinned

3 TB. canola oil

1 cup green beans, trimmed

4 cups mixed salad greens torn into bite-size pieces

2 TB. toasted sesame seeds

1. To make dressing: in a small bowl, mix sesame oil, orange rind, orange juice, mustard, tarragon, and season to taste with salt and pepper. Set aside.

2. Cut salmon into bite-size pieces. Heat canola oil in a skillet and sauté salmon pieces for 3–4 minutes, until lightly browned and tender inside.

3. While salmon is cooking, cook green beans in boiling salted water for 5–6 minutes, until tender yet still slightly crisp.

4. Arrange mixed salad greens on serving plates. Drain beans and add to the plates. Spoon salmon onto the plates. Sprinkle with toasted sesame seeds. Top with desired amount of dressing. Serve while warm.

Tasty Tidbits _____

You can purchase sesame seeds already toasted or toast them yourself. To toast, heat a skillet over medium heat. Add sesame seeds and stir for 2–3 minutes until fragrant and browned.

Shrimp and Mint Asian Salad

Ginger, coconut milk, and fish sauce impart a hot, sweet, and musky flavor to the shrimp.

12 large raw shrimp	1 tsp. sugar
1 TB. olive oil	1 tsp. minced garlic
1 TB. fish sauce	2 fresh red chiles, seeded and finely chopped
1 TB. fresh lime juice	
3 TB. coconut milk	⅛ tsp. ground black pepper
1 (1-inch) piece of fresh ginger, peeled and grated	2 TB. fresh mint leaves
	4 cups butter lettuce leaves, torn in bite-size pieces

1. Peel shrimp, leaving tails.

2. Heat olive oil in a large skillet and sauté shrimp until they turn pink.

3. Mix fish sauce, lime juice, coconut milk, ginger, sugar, garlic, chiles, and pepper together in a small bowl for dressing.

4. Toss warm shrimp with dressing and mint leaves. Serve shrimp mixture on bed of green lettuce leaves. Top with desired amount of dressing.

Yields 12 shrimp and 4 cups lettuce

Prep time: 15 minutes

Cook time: 5 minutes

Serving size: 3 shrimp and 1 cup lettuce

Each serving:

Salad:

Glycemic index: low

Glycemic load: 2

Calories: 108

Protein: 18 grams

Carbohydrates: <1 gram

Fiber: 2 grams

Fat: 4 grams

Saturated fat: <1 gram

Salad dressing per tablespoon:

Glycemic index: very low

Glycemic load: 0

Calories: 10

Carbohydrates: <1 gram

Fat: 1 gram

Saturated fat: <1 gram

Chicken, Pear, Walnut Salad with Asiago

Yields 12 cups salad
Prep time: 15 minutes
Cook time: none
Serving size: 2 cups salad
Each serving:
Salad:
Glycemic index: low
Glycemic load: 3
Calories: 221
Protein: 16 grams
Carbohydrates: 10 grams
Fiber: 3 grams
Fat: 13 grams
Saturated fat: 1 gram
Salad dressing per table-spoon:
Glycemic index: very low
Glycemic load: 0
Calories: 72
Carbohydrates: 0 grams
Fat: 8 grams
Saturated fat: 1 gram

A mild and sweet blend of lettuce and pears spiked with the sharp tang of Asiago cheese.

¼ cup olive oil

2 TB. white wine vinegar

⅛ tsp. freshly ground black pepper

8 cups torn Bibb lettuce leaves

2 cups cooked chicken breast, shredded

2 medium-size ripe pears, cored and cut into ½-inch cubes

¾ cup toasted walnut halves

⅓ cup shaved Asiago cheese

1. To make dressing, combine olive oil, white wine vinegar and pepper in a jar with a tight-fitting lid and shake to blend.

2. Place lettuce in a large salad bowl. Add chicken, pears, and walnuts. Top with desired amount of dressing and toss gently.

3. Top with Asiago cheese and toss gently. Serve at once.

Tasty Tidbits

Asiago cheese is an Italian cheese that's reminiscent of sharp cheddar and Parmesan.

Chapter 12

Beef Main Dishes

In This Chapter

- ◆ Beef is a good food for weight loss
- ◆ Satisfying low-glycemic beef dishes
- ◆ Lowering fat content

Beef satisfies our hunger for power food. Beef contains high-quality protein, a high-concentration of B vitamins and important minerals, essential fatty acids, and CLA—conjugated linoleic acid.

Our beef recipes deliver lean meat, even from fatty cuts of beef:

- ◆ Cut off visible fat from the meat before cooking.

- ◆ After browning meats, pour off the fat from the skillet or saucepan and discard.

- ◆ After roasting, spoon fat from pan juices before making sauces and gravies. Discard fat.

Long roasting times at low temperatures make chuck roasts and other fatty cuts of meat very tender and render out most of the fat into the pan juices, which you can discard. Use lean ground beef in recipes that call for ground beef.

Sweet Potatoes and Beef Oven Roast

Yields 1 (3-lb.) pot roast and vegetables
Prep time: 20 minutes
Cook time: 1³/₄ hours, plus 15–20 minutes
Serving size: 3 oz. beef and ¹/₈ vegetables
Each serving:
Glycemic index: low
Glycemic load: 10
Calories: 225
Protein: 21 grams
Carbohydrates: 10 grams
Fiber: 2 grams
Fat: 11 grams
Saturated fat: 3 grams

Sweet potatoes, cinnamon, and ginger add sweetness and heat to this juicy pot roast.

2 TB. olive oil

1 (3-lb.) boneless beef chuck roast

1 (14-oz.) can natural beef broth

1 TB. Worcestershire sauce

1 tsp. salt

½ tsp. freshly ground black pepper

3 medium sweet potatoes, peeled and cut into ½-inch slices

1 (14-oz.) pkg. frozen whole green beans

3 carrots, washed and sliced

1 large onion, peeled and cut into wedges

¼ tsp. ground cinnamon

1 inch of ginger root, diced

1 cup water

1 tsp. honey

1 TB. cornstarch

1. In a large skillet with a lid, heat olive oil at medium-high heat. Add roast and brown. Drain fat and discard. Pour broth and Worcestershire sauce over roast. Add salt and pepper. Bring to a boil. Reduce heat and simmer, covered, for 1³/₄ hours.

2. Add potatoes, beans, carrots, onion, cinnamon, and ginger root. Return to boiling, then reduce heat. Simmer, covered, 15 to 20 minutes or until meat and vegetables are tender.

3. Transfer meat and vegetables to a platter. For gravy, skim off fat. Add water and honey to skillet. Stir in cornstarch. Cook and stir over medium heat until thickened. Serve with roast and vegetables.

Variation: For less fat and calories, use a 3 oz. meat portion instead of 6 oz. meat portion.

Home-Cooked Goodness

Sweet potatoes aren't just a healthier substitute for white potatoes. They also add a delicious light, sweet flavor to meat and seafood.

Meatloaf with Pine Nuts

Oranges and green chiles add a hot, tangy citrus sweetness.

¾ lb. lean (95% fat-free) ground beef

¼ lb. extra-lean ground pork

1 (11-oz.) can Mandarin oranges, drained

1 (4.5-oz.) can diced green chiles, drained

2 TB. pine nuts

1 egg, lightly beaten

1 tsp. chili powder

½ tsp. salt

½ cup fruit salsa (See Chapter 9 for suggestions.)

1. Preheat the oven to 350°F.

2. In a mixing bowl, mix beef and pork together. Stir in oranges, green chiles, pine nuts, egg, chili powder, and salt. Press into a 9×5×4-inch loaf pan. Bake for 1 hour. Drain excess fat from pan while warm. Serve with heated fruit salsa.

Yields 1 lb. meatloaf
Prep time: 10 minutes
Cook time: 1 hour
Serving size: 2½ oz. meatloaf
Each serving:
Glycemic index: low
Glycemic load: 2
Calories: 173
Protein: 20 grams
Carbohydrates: 8 grams
Fiber: 1 gram
Fat: 6.7 grams
Saturated fat: 2.25 grams

Pomegranate Flank Steak

This steak is flavored with pomegranate and soy sauce.

2 lbs. lean flank steak

3 TB. red wine vinegar

¼ cup unsweetened pomegranate juice

3 TB. soy sauce

3 TB. olive oil

1 tsp. minced garlic

1 tsp. chili powder

1. In a large plastic resealable food storage bag, place steak, vinegar, pomegranate juice, soy sauce, olive oil, garlic, and chili powder.

2. Marinate at room temperature for 3–4 hours. If you need to marinate longer, refrigerate.

3. Heat the grill on high and cook steak to your preferred level of doneness, reserving marinade.

4. Cook marinade in a small saucepan to reduce sauce by half. Serve sauce with thinly sliced steak.

Yields 2 lbs. steak plus sauce
Prep time: 3–4 hours
Cook time: 15 minutes
Serving size: 3 oz. steak
Each serving:
Glycemic index: very low
Glycemic load: 0
Calories: 210
Protein: 23 grams
Carbohydrates: 1 gram
Fiber: 0 grams
Fat: 14 grams
Saturated fat: 4 grams

Spaghetti Squash with Meat Sauce

Enjoy the herby garlic and oregano flavors of spaghetti meat sauce in each squash half.

Yields 1 stuffed spaghetti squash
Prep time: 15 minutes
Cook time: 1 hour
Serving size: ¼ squash plus filling
Each serving:
Glycemic index: low
Glycemic load: 4
Calories: 153
Protein: 10 grams
Carbohydrates: 15 grams
Fiber: 3 grams
Fat: 5.9 grams
Saturated fat: 1.6 grams

½ lb. extra-lean (95% fat-free) ground beef

1 small onion, finely chopped

1 tsp. minced garlic

1 TB. olive oil

½ green pepper, finely chopped

½ cup sliced mushrooms

1 (16-oz.) can stewed tomatoes, chopped

½ tsp. basil

½ tsp. oregano

¼ tsp. salt

⅛ tsp. freshly ground black pepper

1 medium spaghetti squash, cut in half, seeds and inner fibers removed

2 TB. shredded Parmesan cheese

1. Preheat the oven to 350°F.

2. Sauté ground beef, onion, and garlic in oil in a large saucepan over medium-high heat until beef is lightly browned. Drain off fat. Stir in green peppers, mushrooms, stewed tomatoes, basil, oregano, salt, and pepper.

3. Place squash halves in an oven baking dish. Fill with beef mixture. Bake 45 minutes or until squash is easily pierced with a fork.

4. Sprinkle halves with Parmesan cheese and return to the oven for 5 minutes.

 Tasty Tidbits _____

Spaghetti squash is a wonderful low-glycemic treat and an excellent substitute for wheat pasta if you're sensitive to wheat or gluten.

Italian Beef Tenderloin

Sweet potatoes balance the rich garlic flavor of the tenderloin.

1 TB. dried Italian seasoning

1 TB. roasted minced garlic

1 tsp. salt

½ tsp. crushed red pepper

3 TB. olive oil

2 lbs. sweet potatoes, cut into 1-inch wedges

2 lbs. beef tenderloin

1 recipe Orange Garlic Topping (see below)

1. Preheat the oven to 425°F.

2. In a small bowl, combine Italian seasoning, garlic, salt, and crushed red pepper. Stir in olive oil. Divide seasoning mixture between two large, re-sealable plastic bags. Place sweet potatoes in one bag; shake to coat potatoes.

3. Place beef in the remaining bag. Shake to coat. In a large skillet, brown beef tenderloin over medium-high heat, turning to brown evenly. Place browned tenderloin in center of a greased roasting pan. Place sweet potato wedges around the pan edges.

4. Roast, uncovered, 30 to 35 minutes for medium-rare (140°F), or 40 to 45 minutes for medium (155°F). Let stand for 5 minutes before carving beef. Spread Orange Garlic Topping recipe on roast before serving.

Yields 8 servings tenderloin

Prep time: 20 minutes

Cook time: 30 to 45 minutes, plus 5 minutes stand time

Serving size: ¼ lb. (4 oz.) beef and ¼ lb. sweet potatoes

Each serving:

Glycemic index: low

Glycemic load: 5

Calories: 342

Protein: 30 grams

Carbohydrates: 15 grams

Fiber: 2 grams

Fat: 18 grams

Saturated fat: 5 grams

Orange Garlic Topping

Yields 8 servings
Prep time: 5 minutes
Cook time: none
Serving size: 6 TB.
Each serving:
Glycemic index: very low
Glycemic load: 0
Calories 2
Protein: 0 grams
Carbohydrates: <1 gram
Fiber: <1 gram
Fat: 0 grams
Saturated fat.: 0 grams

Spread the parsley, orange, and garlic topping on this succulent tenderloin to enhance the Italian accent. This topping has no glycemic value, and virtually no calories or fat.

¼ **cup chopped fresh parsley**   **2 cloves garlic, minced**

2 tsp. finely shredded orange peel, or 1 tsp. dried orange peel

1. Stir parsley, orange peel, and garlic together in a small bowl.

2. Spread on roast before serving.

Home-Cooked Goodness

Re-sealable food storage bags work well as containers for marinating meat and for shaking a combination of spices onto meats or vegetables.

Beef and Ale

Ale imparts a rich flavor and intensifies the meaty taste of chuck steak.

3 TB. olive oil

2 lbs. chuck steak, cut into 1½-inch pieces

1 medium onion, sliced

1 cup carrots, thinly sliced

2 cups celery stalks, thinly sliced

1 tsp. mustard powder

1 tsp. tomato paste

1×3-inch strip orange rind

2½ cups Guinness or other dark ale

Salt and freshly ground black pepper

2 tsp. *bouquet garni* (parsley, bay leaf, thyme)

Yields 2 lbs. meat plus 4 cups vegetables and gravy

Prep time: 30 minutes
Cook time: 2–3 hours
Serving size: 3 oz. meat and ⅓ cup vegetables

Each serving:
Glycemic index: low
Glycemic load: 3
Calories: 216
Protein: 21 grams
Carbohydrates: 5 grams
Fiber: 1 gram
Fat: 12 grams
Saturated fat: 4 grams

1. Heat 1 tablespoon of oil over medium heat in a large saucepan. Add beef and sauté until lightly browned. Transfer into a bowl. Discard any fat in pan.

2. Add remaining 2 tablespoons oil to the pan and sauté sliced onion until browned, adding thinly sliced carrot and celery toward the end.

3. Stir in mustard, tomato paste, orange rind, ale, and seasoning, then add bouquet garni and bring to a boil.

4. Return meat, and any juice in bowl, to the pan. Make sure meat is covered, and add water if necessary. Cover pan with a tight-fitting lid and cook for 2 to 2½ hours over medium-low heat, until meat is very tender.

def•i•ni•tion

Bouquet garni is the French cooking designation for a combination of the three herbs: parsley, bay leaf, and thyme. You can purchase a premixed version at the grocery store, or blend your own with each recipe.

Paprika Beef with Roasted Peppers

Paprika is a sweet, warm pepper that imparts a red glow to this tender beef dish.

Yields 1½ lbs. beef and 2 cups vegetables

Prep time: 30 minutes

Cook time: 3 hours

Serving size: 3 oz. beef and ⅓ cup vegetables

Each serving:

Glycemic index: low

Glycemic load: 1

Calories: 216

Protein: 22 grams

Carbohydrates: 5 grams

Fiber: 1 gram

Fat: 13 grams

Saturated fat: 5 grams

2 TB. olive oil	1 (14-oz.) can chopped tomatoes
1½ lbs. chuck steak, cut into 1½-inch pieces	¼ tsp. salt
2 onions, chopped	¼ tsp. freshly ground black pepper
1 garlic clove, crushed	2 red bell peppers, halved, seeded, cut in strips
1 TB. flour	⅔ cup low-fat sour cream
1 TB. paprika, plus extra to garnish	

1. Preheat the oven to 275°F.

2. In a large ovenproof baking dish over medium heat, add oil and brown chuck steak in batches. Remove meat from the baking dish with a slotted spoon to a plate and set aside.

3. Add onions and garlic to the baking dish. Sauté until softened but not browned. Stir in flour and paprika and continue cooking for 1–2 minutes, stirring continuously to prevent sticking.

4. Return meat and any juice that has collected on the plate to the baking dish. Add chopped tomatoes, salt, and black pepper. Bring to a boil while stirring continuously, then cover with a tight-fitting lid and bake in the oven for 2½ hours.

5. Add peppers to the baking dish and bake for 15–30 more minutes, or until meat is tender. Remove from the oven.

6. Stir in sour cream. Arrange on a serving platter and sprinkle with a little paprika.

Grilled Steak with Horseradish Sauce

Horseradish imparts a tangy, warming flavor to beef, giving you a creamy steak with a kick.

2 lbs. extra-lean beef rib-eye or sirloin steaks

1 TB. olive oil

1 tsp. dried rosemary, crushed

½ tsp. coarse sea salt or kosher salt

1 recipe Horseradish Sauce (see below, calories and fat calculated separately)

Sliced radishes (optional)

1. Preheat the grill to medium-high.

2. Cut visible fat from steaks. Brush steaks with olive oil; sprinkle with rosemary and salt. Grill until steaks are cooked to your taste preference.

3. Serve with horseradish sauce below. Garnish with sliced radishes (if using).

Yields 2 lbs. meat
Prep time: 10 minutes
Cook time: 35–40 minutes
Serving size: ¼ pound steak
Each serving:
Glycemic index: very low
Glycemic load: 0
Calories: 186
Protein: 28 grams
Carbohydrates: <1 gram
Fiber: 0 grams
Fat: 8 grams
Saturated fat: 1.98 grams

Home-Cooked Goodness

Horseradish uniquely complements beef—roasts, burgers, steak—and adds zip to your meat dishes.

Horseradish Sauce

Horseradish sauce adds zest to beef roasts and burgers.

¼ cup mayonnaise

1 TB. prepared horseradish

1 TB. chopped parsley

⅛ tsp. freshly ground black pepper

Stir together mayonnaise, horseradish, parsley, and pepper in a small bowl. Serve desired amount with beef or vegetables.

Yields ¼ cup sauce
Prep time: 10 minutes
Cook time: none
Serving size: 1 TB. sauce
Glycemic index: very low
Glycemic load: 0
Calories: 99
Carbohydrates: 0 grams
Fiber: <1 gram
Fat: 11 grams
Saturated fat: 1.5 grams

Pot Roast with Potatoes and Carrots

Yields 2½–3 lbs. pot roast
Prep time: 30 minutes
Cook time: 1¾ hours
Serving size: 3 oz. meat and 1 cup vegetables
Each serving:
Glycemic index: low
Glycemic load: 6
Calories: 263
Protein: 25 grams
Carbohydrates: 12 grams
Fiber: 1 gram
Fat: 14 grams
Saturated fat: 4 grams

A splash of red wine in the pan sauces adds a bold, elegant flavor to the beef and vegetables.

1 (2.5-lb. to 3-lb.) boneless beef chuck roast

¼ tsp. freshly ground black pepper

3 TB. olive oil

2 large onions, cut into ¾-inch slices

¾ cup water

¼ cup red wine vinegar

1 tsp. dried thyme, crushed

¼ tsp. salt

1 lb. small red potatoes

1 lb. carrots, cut in 2-inch pieces

2 stalks celery, cut in 1-inch pieces

2 tsp. butter

¼ cup red wine

1. Trim fat from roast. Sprinkle with pepper. Heat olive oil at medium heat in a large saucepan and brown roast. Remove roast and add onions, cooking until browned. Return roast to the saucepan. Combine water, vinegar, thyme, and salt. Pour over roast and onions. Bring to boil, then reduce heat. Simmer, covered, for 1 hour.

2. Peel a strip of skin from center of each potato. Add potatoes, carrots, and celery to the pan. Return to boiling, then reduce heat. Simmer, covered, for 45 to 55 minutes more or until roast and vegetables are tender. Transfer meat and vegetables to a serving platter, reserving juices in the saucepan. Keep meat and vegetables warm.

3. To make sauce, skim fat off reserved juices. Heat saucepan and stir in butter, scraping edges and bottom of pot. Add wine and cook, stirring constantly, for 2–3 minutes to evaporate alcohol.

4. To serve, spoon sauce over roast and vegetables.

Variation: Substitute brandy or white wine for the red wine. For less fat, omit butter, decrease olive oil to 1 tablespoon, and decrease meat portion to 3 ounces.

Pot Roast with Fruit and Vegetables

Fruit gives this pot roast a sweet flavor and an aromatic finish.

1 (2.5-lb.) boneless beef chuck pot roast

2 cloves garlic, minced

1 tsp. dried sage, crushed

¼ tsp. cayenne

½ tsp. black pepper

¼ cup red wine or ¼ cup water

1 large onion, cut into thin wedges

1 cup dried pitted prunes, halved

1 lb. apples, cored and cut in thick wedges

1 lb. carrots, peeled and cut in 2-inch pieces

1 TB. butter

2 TB. olive oil

1 cup red wine or water

1 TB. red wine vinegar

Yields 1 pot roast and 6 cups vegetables and fruit	
Prep time: 30 minutes	
Cook time: 3½ hours	
Serving size: ¼ pound meat with ½ cup vegetables and fruit	
Each serving:	
Glycemic index: low	
Glycemic load: 6	
Calories: 314	
Protein: 29 grams	
Carbohydrates: 18 grams	
Fiber: 15 grams	
Fat: 14 grams	
Saturated fat: 4.2 grams	

1. Preheat the oven to 275°F.

2. Trim fat from roast. Place in a large covered baking pan.

3. In a small bowl, stir together garlic, sage, cayenne, and black pepper. Pat garlic-spice mixture on the surface of the roast. Pour ¼ cup red wine or ¼ cup water over roast; add onion. Cover and bake for 2½ hours.

4. Add onion, prunes, apples, and carrots to roast. Cover and bake for 1 hour or until carrots and apples are tender. Remove roast, fruit, and vegetables to a serving platter.

5. For sauce, skim fat from the baking pan. Add butter and oil and stir with a spoon to loosen pan drippings. Add wine or water and vinegar and cook, stirring, constantly for 2–3 minutes. Serve sauce over roast, vegetables, and fruits.

Variation: For less fat and calories, omit butter, decrease oil to 1 tablespoon, and decrease meat portion to 3 ounces.

 Tasty Tidbits

Adding wine to the pot further tenderizes the meat and enhances the flavor of the apples and prunes.

Pepper Steaks with Madeira Cream Sauce

Steaks have a luxurious flavor with extra pepper and sweet wine sauce.

Yields 4 steaks	

Prep time: 15 minutes, plus 3 hours marinade time

Cook time: 15 minutes

Serving size: 1 steak plus sauce

Each serving:

Glycemic index: very low

Glycemic load: 0

Calories: 418

Protein: 36 grams

Carbohydrates: 1 gram

Fiber: 0 grams

Fat: 27.5 grams

Saturated fat: 14 grams

4 (5-oz.) sirloin or rib-eye steaks	**1 TB. mixed dried peppercorns (green, pink, and black)**
1 TB. olive oil	**1 tsp. olive oil**
1 garlic clove, crushed	**6 TB. water**
4 TB. Madeira wine or Sherry	**⅔ cup heavy cream**
	⅛ tsp. salt

1. Trim visible fat from steaks. Place in a gallon-size plastic food-storage bag. Add olive oil, garlic, and Madeira wine or sherry. Seal and marinate in a cool place for at least 4–6 hours, or overnight for more intense flavor. Turn the bag every couple hours.

2. When ready to cook, remove steaks from the bag, reserving marinade. Finely crush peppercorns with a coffee grinder or mortar and pestle. Press evenly onto both sides of steaks.

3. Brush oil in a large heavy skillet and heat on high.

4. Add steaks to the skillet and cook to your taste preference, turning once. Allow about 2 minutes cooking time per side for a rare steak, or 3 minutes per side for medium. Remove steaks from the skillet and keep warm.

5. Add reserved marinade and water to the skillet and bring to a slow boil. Reduce sauce to half its original volume.

6. Add heavy cream to pan. Add salt and stir until sauce has thickened slightly. Top pepper steaks with sauce and serve.

Variation: For less fat, use a low-fat cream (fat-free half-and-half) in place of the heavy cream. Results: 283 calories, 12.5 grams, 3.5 grams saturated fat.

Fiesta Tamale Pie

Chiles and cheese give this meat pie a zesty Southwestern flavor.

¼ cup finely chopped onion

1 TB. olive oil

1 lb. extra-lean ground beef

1 TB. salt

½ tsp. freshly ground black pepper

1 (4-oz.) can diced mild green chiles

1 (16-oz.) can black beans

1 (16-oz.) can corn

1 (4.5-oz.) can chopped ripe olives

1 (1 lb. 12-oz.) can tomatoes

1 cup coarse cornmeal

½ cup grated cheddar cheese

Yields 12 servings pie
Prep time: 10 minutes
Cook time: 40 minutes
Serving size: ¹/₁₂ recipe
Each serving:
Glycemic index: low
Glycemic load: 11
Calories: 240
Protein: 17 grams
Carbohydrates: 24 grams
Fiber: 4 grams
Fat: 6.5 grams
Saturated fat: 1.96 grams

1. Preheat the oven to 350°F.

2. Heat a skillet over medium-high heat and brown onion in olive oil until translucent. Add lean ground beef and brown. Drain. Add salt and pepper.

3. Add green chiles, beans, corn, olives, and tomatoes. Simmer for 5 minutes.

4. Mix cornmeal in simmered ingredients and pour into a 9×13-inch baking dish. Sprinkle with grated cheese.

5. Bake, uncovered, 15 to 20 minutes at 350°F or until cheese is melted.

Home-Cooked Goodness

Store leftovers in glass containers and refrigerate. Eat within 4 days. Reheat in the microwave oven or a traditional oven. If you must store in plastic containers, reheat in glass or ceramic containers without plastic wrapping.

Beef Kabobs

Tender beef is flavored with a mustard lemon marinade.

2 tsp. minced garlic	**2 Bermuda onions**
1 cup olive oil	**1 green bell pepper**
¼ cup soy sauce	**1 red bell pepper**
¼ cup Dijon mustard	**1 yellow bell pepper**
¼ cup fresh lemon juice	**1 lb. small to medium mushrooms**
1 tsp. freshly ground black pepper	**2 pints cherry tomatoes**
3 lbs. sirloin tip beef roast	

Yields 16 kabobs

Prep time: 20 minutes, plus 6 hours marinate time

Cook time: 10 minutes

Serving size: 2 kabobs

Each serving:

Glycemic index: very low

Glycemic load: 0

Calories: 376

Protein: 43 grams

Carbohydrates: 6 grams

Fiber: 1 gram

Fat: 20 grams

Saturated fat: 4.4 grams

1. In a large bowl, mix together garlic, oil, soy sauce, mustard, lemon juice, and black pepper.

2. Cut beef into 1½-inch cubes. Add to the bowl. Stir to cover meat on all sides. Cover and marinate in the refrigerator for 6 hours or longer, stirring occasionally.

3. Cut onions and peppers into large pieces that can be skewered. Cut stems off mushrooms. Assemble skewers, alternating meat with vegetables, including tomatoes.

4. Grill meat over medium-high heat about 3 minutes per side, basting with marinade while cooking.

Variation: For lower fat and calories, decrease olive oil and replace its volume with lemon juice and soy sauce.

Home-Cooked Goodness

Use stainless-steel skewers for these kabobs to support the weight of the beef and vegetables.

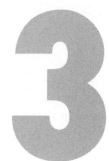

Pork, Lamb, and Veal Main Dishes

In This Chapter

◆ Cooking with pork, lamb, and veal

◆ Sweet and savory tastes

◆ Varying your meats for appetizing tastes

Pork, lamb, and veal offer you the high-quality protein you need to boost your metabolism, lose weight, and keep your energy high. All while they offer you distinct and sometimes unexpected tastes—which you'll find in the mouthwatering recipes in this chapter.

Creole Pork Chops

Yields 6 pork chops
Prep time: 15 minutes
Cook time: 1½ hours
Serving size: 1 pork chop
Each serving:
Glycemic index: low
Glycemic load: 4
Calories: 272
Protein: 30 grams
Carbohydrates: 8 grams
Fiber: 0 grams
Fat: 13.4 grams (used 4 oz. lean chops)
Saturated fat: 6 grams

This Creole recipe gives you the fragrant hot and tangy Gulf Coast flavor of tomatoes, mustard, and ginger.

6 thick (about ¾-inch) center-cut lean pork chops, about 4 oz. each

1 TB. olive oil

¼ cup tomato paste

1⅓ cups water

¼ cup cider vinegar

1½ tsp. dry mustard

1½ tsp. Worcestershire sauce

2 TB. brown sugar

½ tsp. celery seed

½ tsp. fresh ginger, grated

2 tsp. flour

1. Trim visible fat from chops.

2. In a large saucepan, heat olive oil and brown chops. Transfer chops to a plate, skim off excess fat from the pan, and discard.

3. In a small bowl, stir together tomato paste, water, vinegar, dry mustard, Worcestershire sauce, brown sugar, celery seed, fresh ginger, and flour to make sauce.

4. Return chops to the pan and add sauce. Simmer gently on low to medium heat 1½ hours, or until chops are cooked to medium or well-done.

def•i•ni•tion

Creole cuisine is named after the original settlers in Louisiana, before it became part of the United States in 1803. It's a blend of **French**, **Spanish**, **African**, and **Native-American** food traditions.

Curried Pork Chops with Apricots

The sweet taste of apricots, raisins, and coconut is spiced up with a hot curry flavor.

4 lean pork loin chops

1 TB. olive oil

1 onion, thinly sliced

2 yellow peppers, seeded and sliced

2 tsp. curry powder

1 cup water

⅓ cup coarsely chopped dried apricots

2 TB. golden raisins

2 TB. whole-grain mustard

2 TB. shredded coconut

Yields 4 pork chops with 2 cups vegetables and fruit
Prep time: 10 minutes
Cook time: 30 minutes
Serving size: 1 pork chop and ½ cup vegetables and fruit
Each serving:
Glycemic index: low
Glycemic load: 5
Calories: 250
Protein: 23 grams
Carbohydrates: 17 grams
Fiber: 2 grams
Fat: 10 grams
Saturated fat: 3 grams

1. Trim excess fat from pork chops. Heat olive oil in a large skillet over medium-high heat. Add pork chops and sauté until lightly browned.

2. Add onions and yellow peppers to the pan and stir over medium heat for 5 minutes. Stir in curry powder.

3. Add water. Stir in apricots, raisins, and mustard. Cover with a tight-fitting lid and simmer for 25–30 minutes until tender.

4. Place pork and vegetables/fruit on a serving platter. Sprinkle with coconut.

Tasty Tidbits

Curry is a golden blend of spices from India that adds heat and spicy fragrance to food.

Garlic Pork Chops

Yields 6 pork chops
Prep time: 10 minutes
Cook time: 40 minutes
Serving size: 1 pork chop
Each serving:
Glycemic index: very low
Glycemic load: 0
Calories: 296
Protein: 28 grams
Carbohydrates: 1 gram
Fiber: 0 grams
Fat: 20 grams (using lean chops plus fat from oil)
Saturated fat: 6 grams

Garlic, sage, and rosemary add a sunny, herbal, Mediterranean flavor to succulent pork.

4 TB. olive oil	**1 tsp. dried sage**
6 (1-inch-thick) lean pork chops, about 4 oz. each	**3 tsp. minced garlic**
	½ tsp. salt
½ cup dry white wine	**¼ tsp. freshly ground black pepper**
1 tsp. dried rosemary, crushed	**2 TB. dry white wine**

1. Heat 3 tablespoons olive oil in a heavy skillet over medium-high heat. Sauté pork chops until browned, about 2 minutes per side.

2. Add ½ cup wine and cook until evaporated.

3. Sprinkle chops with rosemary, sage, garlic, salt, and pepper.

4. Reduce heat, cover the skillet, and cook 25 minutes, turning once. Remove chops to serving platter.

5. Add 2 tablespoons wine and remaining 1 tablespoon olive oil to the skillet. Stir to blend pan juices. Pour over chops. Serve.

Caribbean Pork Tenderloin

Rich sweetness accented with garlic and pepper on tender pork.

2 TB. dark molasses

2 TB. dark rum

1 tsp. minced garlic

1 tsp. salt

½ tsp. freshly ground black
pepper

½ tsp. black peppercorns

½ tsp. ground cloves

¾ cup fresh lime juice

3 lbs. lean pork tenderloin

½ cup water

Yields 3 lbs. tenderloin and 1 cup sauce
Prep time: 15 minutes, plus overnight marinate time
Cook time: 20–25 minutes
Serving size: 4 oz. pork and 2 TB. sauce
Each serving: Glycemic index: low Glycemic load: <1 Calories: 188 Protein: 29 grams Carbohydrates: <1 gram Fiber: 0 grams Fat: 6 grams Saturated fat: 2 grams

1. In a large glass baking dish, stir together molasses, rum, garlic, salt, pepper, peppercorns, cloves, and lime juice. Add pork to the dish and marinate in the refrigerator overnight, turning occasionally.

2. Preheat the grill to medium-high. Grill pork until a meat thermometer inserted into center registers 170°. Remove from the grill to a serving platter.

3. In a small saucepan over high heat, cook marinade and water to boiling. Continue boiling gently for 2–3 minutes until sauce is reduced.

4. Slice pork and serve with sauce.

Tasty Tidbits ⎯⎯⎯⎯⎯⎯⎯⎯⎯⎯⎯⎯⎯⎯⎯⎯⎯⎯

Increase the heat in this pork dish by adding more peppercorns to the marinade.

Pork Loin with Celery

Celery, herbes de Provence, and dry white wine impart a French country flavor—earthy and robust.

3 TB. olive oil	**⅔ cup water**
2¼ lbs. boned, rolled loin of pork, trimmed of fat	**1 celery head, stalks cut into 1-inch lengths**
1 onion, chopped	**⅔ cup heavy cream**
1 tsp. *herbes de Provence*	**1 TB. lemon juice**
⅔ cup dry white wine	

1. Heat 3 tablespoons olive oil over medium-high heat in a large skillet with a lid. Brown pork. Transfer pork to a plate.

2. Add onion to the skillet and cook until softened but not browned. Add herbes de Provence. Place pork on top and add any juice from the plate. Pour wine and water over pork. Cover, reduce heat, and simmer gently for 30 minutes.

3. Turn pork, arrange celery around it, cover, and cook for 40 minutes, until pork and celery are tender. Transfer pork and celery to a serving plate, cover, and keep warm.

4. Spoon fat from pan juices and discard fat. Stir in cream, bring to a boil, and add lemon juice.

5. Slice pork. Serve cream sauce separately.

Variation: For lower fat, eliminate heavy cream and lemon juice. Instead, serve pork with pan juices. Results: 254 calories, 18 grams fat, 6 grams saturated fat.

Yields 2¼ lbs. pork with 1 cup cooked celery

Prep time: 15 minutes
Cook time: 1½ hours
Serving size: 4 oz. meat and ⅛ vegetables

Each serving:
Glycemic index: low
Glycemic load: <1
Calories: 321
Protein: 20 grams
Carbohydrates: 2 grams
Fiber: <1 gram
Fat: 25 grams
Saturated fat: 10.5 grams

---

def•i•ni•tion

Herbes de Provence is a mixture of herbs that usually contains rosemary, marjoram, basil, bay leaf, thyme, and sometimes lavender flowers. You can purchase it already mixed from the grocery store spice section. It's used in many recipes from the south of France.

Pork Bites with Apples

The tangy, tart apples give these pork bites zest and attitude.

2 TB. olive oil

1¼ lbs. lean pork loin, cut into bite-size pieces

1 onion, coarsely chopped

2 tsp. grated lemon rind

1 cup apple juice

⅔ cup water

2 crisp eating apples, such as Granny Smith, cored and sliced

3 TB. chopped fresh parsley

Yields 1¼ lbs. pork and 1 cup apples	
Prep time: 10 minutes	
Cook time: 35 minutes	
Serving size: 4 oz. pork and ⅕ cup apples	
Each serving:	
Glycemic index: low	
Glycemic load: 6	
Calories: 320	
Protein: 28 grams	
Carbohydrates: 16 grams	
Fiber: 1 gram	
Fat: 16 grams	
Saturated fat: 4 grams	

1. Heat olive oil in a large skillet over medium-high heat. Brown pork. Transfer pork to a platter.

2. Add onions to the pan, and brown lightly. Remove onions to the platter and drain fat from the skillet. Return to heat and stir in lemon rind, apple juice, and water and boil for about 3 minutes. Return pork and onions to the skillet and cook over low to medium heat for about 25 minutes or until tender.

3. Add apples to the pan and cook for 5 minutes. Transfer pork, onions, and apples to a warmed serving dish. Sprinkle with parsley.

Home-Cooked Goodness

Serve with small boiled red potatoes and a green vegetable like beans, asparagus, or peas. This dish is delicious reheated and served in lettuce wraps.

Posole Pork Stew

A thick, spicy stew made with hominy and bold Southwestern seasonings.

Yields 12 cups stew
Prep time: 30 minutes
Cook time: 2 hours
Serving size: 1½ cups stew
Each serving:
Glycemic index: low
Glycemic load: 12
Calories: 380
Protein: 34 grams
Carbohydrates: 25 grams
Fiber: 4 grams
Fat: 16 grams
Saturated fat: 6 grams

2 lbs. lean pork shoulder, cut into 1-inch cubes

1 tsp. salt

¼ tsp. freshly ground black pepper

1 tsp. ground cumin

1 tsp. chili powder

1 TB. fresh chopped cilantro

1½ cups water

2 medium onions, 1 finely chopped, 1 diced

2 tsp. minced garlic

2 (30-oz.) cans hominy, drained and rinsed

1 (4.5-oz.) can diced green chiles

1 cup chopped fresh tomatoes

1. In a large, heavy saucepan with lid, combine pork, salt, pepper, cumin, chili powder, and cilantro. Add water. Over high heat, bring to a boil. Skim off any foam or fat that rises to surface.

2. Reduce heat to medium-low. Add onion and garlic. Cover and simmer for 1 hour.

3. Add hominy, and simmer, uncovered, until pork is tender—about 50 minutes. Add more water if needed.

4. Remove from heat. Posole should be thick. Stir in green chiles and tomatoes. Serve.

Tasty Tidbits

Posole is delicious served the next day after the flavors have had time to blend. Serve with a salad of tomatoes, avocado slices, cucumbers, and green bell peppers.

Cornmeal-Crusted Pork

Pork sautéed with fresh vegetables has a mild flavor enhanced with fresh parsley.

½ cup coarsely ground yellow cornmeal	2 cups trimmed fresh green beans
1 egg, lightly beaten	2 sweet red peppers, sliced
1 TB. water	1 medium zucchini, sliced
1 lb. lean pork tenderloin, cut into ½-inch slices	¼ tsp. salt
2 TB. olive oil	¼ tsp. freshly ground black pepper
	2 TB. chopped fresh parsley

1. Place cornmeal in a shallow dish. In another shallow dish, mix egg with water. Dip pork slices into egg mixture and then into cornmeal to coat.

2. Heat oil in a large skillet over medium heat. Add pork. Cook for 2 minutes per side, or until no pink remains. Transfer to a platter.

3. Add beans, red peppers, and zucchini to skillet; sauté for 6 minutes or until tender. Season with salt and pepper. Transfer to platter with pork and toss. Sprinkle with parsley and serve.

Yields 1 lb. pork and 4 cups vegetables

Prep time: 20 minutes
Cook time: 10 minutes
Serving size: 4 oz. pork and 1 cup vegetables

Each serving:
Glycemic index: low
Glycemic load: <1
Calories: 321
Protein: 30 grams
Carbohydrates: 12 grams
Fiber: 3 grams
Fat: 17 grams
Saturated fat: 3 grams

Chinese Pork with Bell Peppers

Enjoy the warm and earthy taste of Chinese stir-fry with an abundance of colorful, fresh vegetables.

Yields 12 oz. pork with 4 cups vegetables
Prep time: 15 minutes plus 30 minutes marinate time
Cook time: 15 minutes
Serving size: 3 oz. pork and 1 cup vegetables
Each serving:
Glycemic index: low
Glycemic load: 11
Calories: 325
Protein: 26 grams
Carbohydrates: 26 grams
Fiber: 2 grams
Fat: 13 grams
Saturated fat: 3 grams

12-oz. lean pork loin, sliced into strips

2 TB. soy sauce

2 TB. sherry (optional)

1 tsp. brown sugar

1 TB. canola oil

1 TB. sesame oil

1 garlic clove, finely chopped

1 TB. grated fresh ginger

1 red bell pepper, seeded and sliced

1 yellow bell pepper, seeded and sliced

1 green bell pepper, seeded and sliced

1 cup snow peas

4 green onions, cut into 2-inch pieces

2 TB. oyster sauce

4 TB. water

1. In a bowl, mix pork strips, soy sauce, sherry (if using), and brown sugar. Cover and marinate for 30 minutes.

2. Heat oils in a wok or a large frying pan and stir-fry garlic and ginger for about 30 seconds. Add peppers, peas, and onions and stir-fry for 3 minutes.

3. Add pork with marinade juices to a wok or frying pan, and stir-fry for another 3–4 minutes.

4. Finally, pour in oyster sauce and water, and stir until sauce has thickened slightly. Serve immediately.

 Tasty Tidbits _____

Turn up the heat in this traditional stir-fry by adding 1 teaspoon chili powder or ground red pepper flakes in step 4.

Pork Ribs Country-Style

Sauerkraut and celery seed lend a sweet-sour flavor to the ribs.

**3 lbs. (12) pork spareribs
(3 oz edible meat/serving)**

½ tsp. celery seeds

¼ tsp. salt

⅛ tsp. pepper

2 large onions, sliced

1 clove garlic, minced

½ cup water

2 (14-oz.) cans of sauerkraut

1. Preheat the oven to 325°F.

2. Place ribs in a large baking dish with a lid. Add celery seeds, salt, pepper, onions, garlic, and water.

3. Cover and bake for 1½ hours.

4. Remove from the oven briefly and skim off fat. Add sauerkraut. Return to the oven, cover, and bake for 30 minutes.

Yields 12 spareribs and 4 cups sauerkraut with onions
Prep time: 10 minutes
Cook time: 2 hours
Serving size: 3 ribs and 1 cup sauerkraut
Each serving:
Glycemic index: very low
Glycemic load: 0
Calories: 255
Protein: 22 grams
Carbohydrates: 8 grams
Fiber: 3 grams
Fat: 15 grams
Saturated fat: 4.8 grams

Tasty Tidbits

Even if you don't usually like sauerkraut, you may change your mind quickly when presented with these succulent ribs.

Texas Barbecued Ribs

Yields 16 ribs

Prep time: 5 minutes

Cook time: 1 hour 15 minutes

Serving size: 4 ribs (3 oz. edible meat each)

Each serving:

Glycemic index: low

Glycemic load: 7

Calories: 324

Protein: 21 grams

Carbohydrates: 15 grams

Fiber: 0 grams

Fat: 20 grams

Saturated fat: 6 grams

Tangy, spicy, sweet, and robustly flavored ribs satisfy on every level.

3 lbs. (about 16) lean pork spareribs

1 onion, finely chopped

1 large garlic clove, minced

½ cup tomato paste

2 TB. orange juice

2 TB. red wine vinegar

1 tsp. prepared mustard

2 TB. honey

Dash of Worcestershire sauce

2 TB. olive oil

¼ tsp. salt

⅛ tsp. black pepper

2 TB. chopped fresh parsley

1. Preheat the oven to 400°F. Place pork spareribs on top level of an oven broiling pan, so the bottom level catches fat drippings. Bake for 20 minutes.

2. Meanwhile, in a saucepan, mix onion, garlic, tomato paste, orange juice, wine vinegar, mustard, honey, Worcestershire sauce, oil, salt, and pepper. Bring to a boil and simmer for about 5 minutes.

3. Remove ribs from the oven. Reduce oven temperature to 350°F. Using half the sauce, baste ribs, and bake for 20 minutes. Turn ribs over, baste with remaining sauce, and cook for 25 minutes.

4. Sprinkle spareribs with parsley before serving. Allow 4 ribs per person. Provide finger bowls for washing sticky fingers.

Home-Cooked Goodness

When cooking fatty meats such as pork ribs, be sure to use a two-level oven broiler or an outdoor grill to catch the rendered fat. This reduces your saturated fat consumption and lets you enjoy some of the tastiest food in the world.

Brats with Sauerkraut

Sauerkraut gives the brats an old-country taste and adds a healthy sour/acid taste to the meal that's mellowed with apple slices.

2 onions, sliced

1 tsp. garlic, minced

2 TB. olive oil

1 (11-oz.) can sauerkraut with liquid

1 small apple, cored and sliced

2 TB. Dijon-style mustard

½ tsp. celery seed

½ tsp. caraway seed

6 low-fat bratwursts

Yields 6 brats with 2 cups vegetables	
Prep time: 10 minutes	
Cook time: 1 hour	
Serving size: 1 brat (3 oz.) and ⅙ sauerkraut	
Each serving:	
Glycemic index: very low	
Glycemic load: 1	
Calories: 336	
Protein: 12 grams	
Carbohydrates: 9 grams	
Fiber: 2 grams	
Fat: 28 grams	
Saturated fat: 8.6 grams	

1. In a large skillet, sauté onions and garlic in olive oil for 8 minutes or until tender.

2. Add sauerkraut with liquid, apple slices, mustard, celery, and caraway seeds. Cover and simmer for 20 minutes.

3. Add brats and simmer for 40 minutes.

4. Slice brats in half lengthwise and crosswise. Serve on sourdough or stone-ground rolls and top with sauerkraut mixture.

Veal with Lemon and Mushrooms

Yields 12 veal scallops servings
Prep time: 10 minutes
Cook time: 10 minutes
Serving size: 2 veal scallops
Each serving:
Glycemic index: low
Glycemic load: <1
Calories: 227
Protein: 21 grams
Carbohydrates: 2 grams
Fiber: <1 gram
Fat: 15 grams
Saturated fat: 4.5 grams

Veal and mushrooms are enhanced by the tart lemon, and taste bright and fresh.

12 small lean veal scallops, ¼-inch thick, 1½ oz. each	3 TB. olive oil
¼ tsp. salt	1½ cups sliced fresh mushrooms
⅛ tsp. freshly ground black pepper	¼ cup fresh lemon juice
2 TB. flour	2 TB. chopped fresh parsley
	1 TB. butter

1. Place veal between sheets of waxed paper. Pound with side of a rolling pin or meat cleaver to make thin. Remove the paper. Dust with salt, pepper, and flour.

2. Heat 3 tablespoons olive oil in a skillet over medium heat and sauté veal until browned, about 2 minutes on each side. Transfer veal to a serving plate. Add mushrooms to the skillet. Sauté until soft and fragrant. Remove from the skillet to a serving plate.

3. Add lemon juice and parsley to the pan. Remove from heat. Add butter, 1 tablespoon at a time, while stirring to blend pan juices with butter and lemon juice. Serve sauce over veal and mushrooms.

Slow-Cooked Lamb and Black Bean Burritos

Lamb seasoned with garlic and cumin and served with peaches gives a fresh twist to this Southwestern-flavored meal.

2½ lbs. lean lamb shoulder, or 2 lbs. boneless lamb leg

1 (15-oz.) can black beans, rinsed and drained

½ cup apple juice

3 cups water

2 small red sweet peppers, sliced

1 small onion, sliced

⅓ cup dry white wine

8 tsp. minced garlic

1 tsp. salt

½ teaspoon cumin

10 corn or flour tortillas

2 peaches, sliced, or 1½ cups frozen sliced peaches, thawed

¼ cup chopped cilantro

Yields 10 servings
Prep time: 35 minutes
Cook time: 4½ or 9 hours
Serving size: 1 burrito
Each serving:
Glycemic index: low
Glycemic load: 18
Calories: 325
Protein: 30 grams
Carbohydrates: 39 grams
Fiber: 5 grams
Fat: 5.4 grams
Saturated fat: 1.9 grams

1. Trim fat from lamb, and cut meat into bite-size strips. In a 3½- or 4-quart slow cooker, stir together meat strips and black beans, apple juice, water, red sweet peppers, onion, wine, garlic, salt, and cumin.

2. Cover and cook on low-heat setting for 9 to 10 hours, or on high-heat setting for 4½ to 5 hours, then drain.

3. Fill tortillas with lamb filling, peach slices, and cilantro.

Home-Cooked Goodness

Using a slow cooker makes this recipe easier than it seems. Add the ingredients to the cooker in the morning, and by dinnertime the burrito filling is ready for you to serve.

Grilled Lamb Chops

Rosemary, garlic, and onions lend an herbed, savory flavor to the lamb.

Yields 8 lamb loin chops
Prep time: 20 minutes
Cook time: 10 to 14 minutes
Serving size: 1 lamb chop (3 oz each)
Each serving:
Glycemic index: very low
Glycemic load: 0
Calories: 174
Protein: 22 grams
Carbohydrates: 0 grams
Fiber: 0 grams
Fat: 9.6 grams
Saturated fat: 2.47 grams

8 (1-inch thick) lean lamb loin chops (3.5 oz. each)

2 TB. red wine vinegar

1 TB. lemon juice

2 tsp. ground mustard

3 TB. olive oil

1 tsp. minced garlic

1 tsp. rosemary

¼ tsp. salt

⅛ tsp. freshly ground black pepper

1 small onion, sliced

1. Place lamb chops in a deep glass bowl.

2. Combine vinegar, lemon juice, mustard, olive oil, garlic, rosemary, salt, pepper, and onions.

3. Grill over medium-hot coals 5 minutes per side for medium-rare (145°F).

Home-Cooked Goodness

Grilling is an easy way to cook year-round—it's fast, easy, and makes clean-up quick. Top the meat with an interesting sauce or salsa, add a salad or vegetable, and you have a superb meal.

Chapter 14

Poultry Main Dishes

In This Chapter

- ◆ Poultry dishes offer many flavors
- ◆ Easy grilling and baking recipes
- ◆ Spices and herbs that dish up flavorful meals

Chicken and turkey are delicately flavored meats that easily pick up the flavors of both subtle and stronger-tasting herbs and spices. The recipes in this chapter offer you many interesting choices and flavors.

You'll find distinctive Mediterranean, Southwestern, and Italian tastes. Other recipes are mild with the flavors of sweet paprika, pistachios, or basil. We've even included a mild mole dish featuring chili powder and bitter-sweet cocoa.

Parmesan Baked Chicken

Your favorite salad dressing adds bold flavor to this simple baked-chicken recipe.

6 (6-oz.) skinless chicken breasts	**½ cup grated Parmesan cheese**
¾ cup regular salad dressing, your choice, not low-fat	**1 tsp. dried parsley flakes**
	⅛ tsp. freshly ground black pepper

1. Preheat the oven to 350°F.

2. Brush chicken breasts with salad dressing. Mix together Parmesan cheese, parsley, and pepper. Dip tops of chicken breasts in Parmesan mixture. Arrange in a baking dish.

3. Bake at 350°F for 1 hour, or until juices run clear when pierced with a fork.

Variations: Suggested salad dressings include Italian, blue cheese, Thousand Island, Asiago Peppercorn, and French.

Yields 6 chicken breasts

Prep time: 15 minutes

Cook time: 1 hour

Serving size: 1 (6-oz.) chicken breast

Each serving:

Glycemic index: very low

Glycemic load: 0

Calories: 332

Protein: 43 grams

Carbohydrates: 3 grams

Fiber: 0 grams

Fat: 16.5 grams

Saturated fat: 3 grams

Home-Cooked Goodness

Vary the taste of this recipe by changing the salad dressing you use. You can even use olive oil and a flavored vinegar. Use a low-fat salad dressing if you would like to lower the amount of fat.

Glycemic Notes

The fat amounts for this recipe are calculated based on the assumption that half of the butter drips into the grill during cooking.

Oven-Baked Mole Chicken

The spices and cocoa add the mild, smoky flavor of mole to this classic baked chicken.

¼ cup Hi-Maize Resistant Starch

¼ cup coarse yellow cornmeal

1 tsp. chili powder

1 tsp. unsweetened baking cocoa powder like Hershey's

½ tsp. cumin

1 cup low-fat yogurt

1 TB. butter, melted

1 chicken, cut into pieces, or 6 chicken breasts skinned

1. In a large bowl, mix together Hi-Maize Resistant Starch, cornmeal, chili powder, cocoa powder, cumin, yogurt, and melted butter. Dip chicken in mixture and place in a baking dish.

2. Bake for 1 hour. Chicken is cooked when juices run clear when pricked with a fork.

Yields 1 chicken, or 6 chicken breasts	
Prep time: 15 minutes	
Cook time: 1 hour	
Serving size: 1 (6-oz.) chicken breast, or ¹⁄₆ chicken	
Each serving:	
Glycemic index: very low	
Glycemic load: 0	
Calories: 249	
Protein: 45 grams	
Carbohydrates: 9 grams	
Fiber: 1 gram	
Fat: 3.65 grams	
Saturated fat: 1.8 grams	

Tasty Tidbits _____

Mole is a chili sauce flavored with bitter chocolate that originated with the pre-Columbian Mexican culture. It's an acquired taste, which is why we offer you this mild variation. You can increase the heat by doubling the chili and cocoa powders.

Chicken with Red Cabbage

Yields 4 pieces chicken with 4 cups vegetables

Prep time: 15 minutes

Cook time: 50 minutes

Serving size: 1 (6-oz.) piece chicken with 1 cup vegetables

Each serving:

Glycemic index: very low

Glycemic load: 0

Calories: 332

Protein: 46 grams

Carbohydrates: 10 grams

Fiber: 8 grams

Fat: 12 grams

Saturated fat: 2.6 grams

Red cabbage with a hint of juniper berries gives chicken an Eastern European flavor.

4 TB. olive oil	**4 juniper berries, crushed**
4 large chicken pieces, skinless, cut in half	**¼ tsp. salt**
1 onion, chopped	**¼ tsp. freshly ground black pepper**
8 cups finely shredded red cabbage	**½ cup red wine**

1. Heat olive oil in a heavy skillet with a lid. Add chicken pieces and brown lightly. Transfer chicken to a plate.

2. Add onion to the skillet. Sauté until soft and light brown. Stir cabbage and juniper berries into the skillet. Cook over medium heat for about 6–7 minutes, stirring once or twice.

3. Stir in salt and pepper. Return chicken to skillet, and spoon cabbage mixture over chicken. Pour in red wine.

4. Cover and cook gently for about 40 minutes until chicken juices run clear and cabbage is very tender.

Home-Cooked Goodness

At first reading, 8 cups red cabbage may seem like way too much, but as it cooks down, the end result will be a scant 1 cup per person. Serve with small red boiled potatoes and a green vegetable such as green beans or broccoli.

Slow-Cooked Creamy Basil Chicken

Tastes like comfort food: creamy and mild with a fresh basil taste.

2 cups mushrooms, sliced

2 medium red and/or yellow sweet peppers, cut into strips

1 large onion, sliced

8 cloves garlic, minced

8 skinless, boneless chicken breast halves

1¼ cups water

1 lb. fresh asparagus spears, trimmed

⅓ cup heavy cream

½ cup fresh basil, chopped

2 cups cooked basmati rice

2 TB. fresh basil, chopped

Yields 8 chicken breasts and 8 cups vegetables
Prep time: 25 minutes
Cook time: 6 hours (low) + 30 minutes (high), or 3½ hours (high)
Serving size: 1 chicken breast, 1 cup vegetables, and ¼ cup rice
Each serving:
Glycemic index: low
Glycemic load: 6
Calories: 329
Protein: 46 grams
Carbohydrates: 15 grams
Fiber: 3 grams
Fat: 9.4 grams
Saturated fat: 2.314 grams

1. In a 5- or 6-quart slow cooker, stir together mushrooms, sweet pepper, onion, and garlic. Place chicken on top mixture in the cooker. Pour water over all.

2. Cover and cook on low-heat setting for 6–7 hours, or on high-heat setting for 3–3½ hours.

3. Cut asparagus into 2- to 3-inch lengths. Turn slow cooker to high-heat setting. Stir in asparagus, cream, and ½ cup fresh basil. Cover. Cook for 30 minutes.

4. Serve chicken, vegetables, and sauce with rice. Garnish with fresh basil.

Variation: For lower fat, use low-fat yogurt in place of the heavy cream. Results: 298 calories, 6 grams fat, 1.7 grams saturated fat.

Tasty Tidbits _____

Cook this dish on low for six hours if you'll be out during the day. Otherwise, you can use the high setting and let it simmer for an afternoon. You'll return to a delicious meal worthy of praise.

Oat-Crusted Chicken with Sage

Crunchy oats flavored with sage and a sage-flavored yogurt top this baked chicken for an herbal delight.

½ cup long-cooking oats	¼ tsp. freshly ground black pepper
3 TB. fresh sage leaves, chopped, or 1½ tsp. dried sage	8 chicken thighs or drumsticks, skinned
½ tsp. salt	3 TB. milk
	½ cup plain yogurt

Yields 8 chicken pieces and ½ cup yogurt sauce

Prep time: 20 minutes

Cook time: 40 minutes

Serving size: 2 pieces chicken (5 oz.) total and 2 TB. sauce

Each serving:

Glycemic index: low

Glycemic load: 4

Calories: 298

Protein: 35 grams

Carbohydrates: 8 grams

Fiber: 1 gram

Fat: 14 grams

Saturated fat: 4.2 grams

1. Preheat the oven to 400°F.

2. Mix oats with 2 tablespoons fresh or 1 teaspoon dried sage, salt, and pepper on a plate. Brush chicken with milk and press into oat mixture to coat evenly.

3. Place chicken in a baking pan. Bake for about 40 minutes, or until juices run clear, not pink, when pierced with a fork.

4. Meanwhile, mix together yogurt and remaining sage and serve with the chicken.

Variation: Substitute 4 (½) chicken breasts for the thighs and drumsticks.

Home-Cooked Goodness

For most recipes, 1 tablespoon of fresh herb delivers the same value of taste as 1 teaspoon dried.

Spicy Chicken Thighs with Green Beans

Sautéed chicken with the bold flavors of coriander, cumin, cinnamon, and chili powder, and served with tangy blue cheese topping.

2 TB. olive oil

1 tsp. ground coriander

1 tsp. ground cumin

½ tsp. salt

½ tsp. ground cinnamon

¼ tsp. chili powder

1¼ lbs. skinless, boneless chicken thighs

1 cup fresh or frozen green beans

1 cup frozen edamame (green soy beans) or lima beans

1 avocado, halved, seeded, peeled, and sliced

3 oz. blue cheese, broken into chunks

¼ cup bottled creamy garlic or Italian vinaigrette salad dressing.

Yields 1¼ lbs. chicken and 3 cups vegetables	
Prep time: 30 minutes	
Cook time: 35 minutes	
Serving size: 4 oz. chicken and ¾ cup vegetables	
Each serving:	
Glycemic index: very low	
Glycemic load: 1	
Calories: 386	
Protein: 30 grams	
Carbohydrates: 8 grams	
Fiber: 3 grams	
fat: 26 grams	
Saturated fat: 9 grams	

1. Heat a skillet over medium heat.

2. In a small bowl, combine oil, coriander, cumin, salt, cinnamon, and chili powder. Brush oil mixture on both sides of chicken thighs.

3. Place chicken in a skillet. Cook about 12–15 minutes, or until chicken is tender and no longer pink, turning once. Transfer chicken to a cutting board. Cut each chicken thigh into 3 pieces.

4. Meanwhile, in a large saucepan over high heat, cook fresh beans in enough boiling water to cover for 10–15 minutes or until crisp-tender. If using frozen beans, cook for 5–10 minutes or until crisp-tender. Remove beans with a slotted spoon. Set aside. Add edamame to boiling water. Cover and cook for 4–6 minutes or until tender. Drain.

5. Arrange chicken, green beans, edamame, avocado, and cheese on salad plates or a platter; top with blue cheese. Drizzle with dressing. Serve immediately.

 Tasty Tidbits

Edamame is the natural form of soybeans—green, crunchy, and delicious in salads and as a vegetable side dish.

Ginger Chicken Drumsticks

Grilled drumsticks marinated and basted with a sweet, ginger-flavored soy sauce mixture.

Yields 8 drumsticks
Prep time: 15 minutes
Cook time: 30–40 minutes
Serving size: 2 (2-oz.) drumsticks
Each serving:
Glycemic index: low
Glycemic load: 1
Calories: 223
Protein: 28 grams
Carbohydrates: 3 grams
Fiber: 0 grams
Fat: 11.1 grams
Saturated fat: 3 grams

8 chicken drumsticks

2 TB. lemon juice

1 TB. dark molasses

1 tsp. fresh ginger, grated

1 TB. soy sauce

½ tsp. freshly ground black pepper

1. Using a sharp knife, slash drumsticks about 3 times through thickest part of flesh. Mix lemon juice, molasses, ginger, soy sauce, and black pepper in a large bowl. Place drumsticks in lemon juice mixture and turn to coat.

2. Heat grill to hot. Cook drumsticks on grill, turning occasionally and basting with lemon juice mixture, until golden and the juices run clear when pierced.

Home-Cooked Goodness _____

When a recipe calls for grilling, you can also cook in the oven on the high broiler setting.

Chicken Stuffed with Ham and Cheese

Swiss cheese and ham lend a tangy, sweet taste to tender chicken breasts topped with parsley.

6 boneless, skinless chicken breast halves

6 slices Swiss cheese (1 oz. each)

6 thin slices lean 5 percent ham (½ oz. each)

¼ cup butter, melted

6 tsp. dried parsley

1. Heat the oven to 375°F.

2. Pound out chicken breasts with meat hammer until breasts are all about the same thickness.

3. Place 1 cheese slice and 1 piece of ham inside each breast. Roll up breast to enclose cheese and ham. Secure with toothpicks.

4. Dip breasts in butter. Sprinkle with parsley.

5. Bake in a covered baking dish for 45–55 minutes.

Yields 6 stuffed chicken breasts	
Prep time: 15 minutes	
Cook time: 45–55 minutes	
Serving size: 1 (6-oz.) chicken breast	
Each serving:	
Glycemic index: very low	
Glycemic load: 0	
Calories: 371	
Protein: 32 grams	
Carbohydrates: 0 grams	
Fiber: 0 grams	
Fat: 27 grams	
Saturated fat: 7 grams	

Home-Cooked Goodness

The combination of ham and cheese is a perennial favorite and the tastes combine well with poultry, salads, and omelets.

Chicken Paprika

Sweet paprika adds a mellow heat to the chicken, accented by a tangy sour cream sauce.

2 TB. olive oil	**2 cups water**
2 medium-size onions, finely chopped	**2 tsp. flour**
	2 cups sour cream
2 tsp. salt	**2 cups cooked basmati rice**
2 TB. sweet paprika	
4 whole boneless skinned chicken breasts, halved (6 oz. per portion)	

1. Heat olive oil in a skillet over medium-high heat. Sauté onions until golden.

2. Sprinkle with salt and paprika and add chicken. Sauté for 3 minutes. Add water. Cover and simmer until tender, about 45 minutes. Remove chicken from the skillet to a side plate.

3. Combine flour with sour cream. Stir mixture into the skillet with a wire whisk to blend thoroughly with pan juices. Add chicken. Heat thoroughly to below boiling point. Do not boil. Serve immediately over rice.

Variation: For lower fat, use olive oil in place of butter, and light sour cream instead of regular. Results: 352 calories, 7 grams fat, 4 grams saturated fat.

Glycemic Notes

Don't overcook the sour cream sauce. Cook just until warm, being sure not to boil. Boiling will curdle the sauce.

Yields 8 chicken breast	
Prep time: 15 minutes	
Cook time: 48 minutes	
Serving size: 1 chicken breast (6 oz.) and 1/4 cup rice	
Each serving:	
Glycemic index: low	
Glycemic load: 6	
Calories: 413	
Protein: 43 grams	
Carbohydrates: 13 grams	
Fiber: 2 grams	
Fat: 21 grams	
Saturated fat: 9 grams	

Greek Lemon Chicken

Oregano and feta give an authentic Greek taste to the tangy, lemon-flavored chicken.

6 whole large chicken breasts (3 oz. each), boned, skinned, and cut in half

1 cup fruity white wine

¼ cup olive oil

¼ cup fresh lemon juice

1 tsp. freshly grated lemon peel

1 tsp. salt

1 tsp. freshly ground black pepper

3 tsp. garlic, minced

3 TB. olive oil

2 TB. butter

2 TB. flour

½ tsp. salt

1 cup milk

2 egg yolks

1 lemon peel, freshly grated

1 tsp. fresh lemon juice

1 tsp. dried oregano

¼ cup fresh parsley, minced

1 cup sour cream

½ cup feta cheese, crumbled

Yields 12 chicken breast halves
Prep time: 30 minutes, plus 12 hours marinate time
Cook time: 45 minutes
Serving size: 1 (3-oz.) chicken breast half
Each serving:
Glycemic index: low
Glycemic load: <1
Calories: 230
Protein: 24 grams
Carbohydrates: 2 grams
Fiber: 0 grams
Fat: 14 grams
Saturated fat: 5.23 grams

1. Place chicken breasts in a plastic resealable bag. In a bowl, combine marinade portions of wine, olive oil, lemon juice, lemon peel, salt, pepper, and garlic. Pour into a resealable bag. Refrigerate for up to 12 hours.

2. Heat olive oil in a skillet and sauté chicken until tender and cooked. Remove from the skillet to a cutting board. Slice and set aside.

3. In a saucepan, melt butter, then blend in flour and salt. Slowly add milk, stirring constantly until thick and smooth. In a small bowl, mix egg yolk, lemon peel, and lemon juice together. Whisk a small amount of flour mixture into egg mixture. Then whisk egg mixture into flour mixture and bring to a gentle boil. Remove from heat. Add oregano and parsley. Stir in sour cream.

4. Serve sliced chicken topped with milk and sour cream mixture. Sprinkle feta cheese on top.

Variation: For lower fat, use olive oil to replace butter, skim milk, light sour cream, and low-fat feta. Results: 190 calories, 8 grams fat, 3.25 grams saturated fat.

Home-Cooked Goodness

The secret to a creamy sauce with no lumps is to whisk a small amount of the flour mixture into the egg mixture first. Then whisk the two sauces together.

Chicken with Pistachios

Chicken flavored with garlic and paprika, and accented with salty oyster sauce and mild pistachios.

Yields 8 chicken breasts, plus 1½ cups sauce
Prep time: 20 minutes
Cook time: 25 minutes
Serving size: 1 (6-oz.) chicken breast and ⅓ cup sauce
Each serving:
Glycemic index: very low
Glycemic load: 0
Calories: 302
Protein: 44 grams
Carbohydrates: <1 gram
Fiber: <1 g
Fat: 14 grams
Saturated fat: 2.26 grams

4 chicken breasts, halved, boned, and skinned

1 tsp. garlic powder

1 tsp. paprika

¼ tsp. salt

⅛ tsp. freshly ground black pepper

3 TB. olive oil

1 cup natural chicken broth

1 tsp. cornstarch

⅓ cup dry red wine

2 TB. oyster sauce

4 green onions, including tops, chopped

¼ cup pistachio nuts, shelled

1. Season chicken breasts with garlic powder, paprika, salt, and pepper.

2. In a skillet over medium-high heat, sauté chicken in olive oil. Cover and cook 20 minutes until tender and thoroughly cooked. Remove chicken to a serving platter.

3. In the skillet, combine chicken broth, cornstarch, wine, and oyster sauce. Heat to boiling and simmer for 10 minutes. Add green onions and ¼ cup pistachios.

4. Serve chicken with sauce on side.

Tasty Tidbits

Oyster sauce lends an oriental flavor to this simple yet elegant chicken recipe.

Chicken Spaghetti

A fragrant chicken sauce imbued with the rich herbal flavors of rosemary, garlic, and fresh mushrooms.

3 full chicken breasts, halved, skinned, and boned

2 whole celery ribs

1 carrot, cut into rounds

1 onion, studded with 2 whole cloves

2 tsp. dried parsley

1 tsp. salt

12 peppercorns

2 TB. butter

2 green peppers, cored, seeded, chopped

1 large onion, chopped

½ pound mushrooms, chopped

2 tsp. dried rosemary

2 cups tomato sauce

2 spaghetti squash, cooked and removed from shell

½ cup grated Parmesan cheese

Yields 8 cups spaghetti
Prep time: 20 minutes
Cook time: 1½ hours
Serving size: 1 cup spaghetti
Each serving:
Glycemic index: very low
Glycemic load: 1
Calories: 229
Protein: 38 grams
Carbohydrates: 8 grams
Fiber: 3 grams
Fat: 5 grams
Saturated fat: 1.5 grams

1. Place chicken breasts in a heavy saucepan. Add whole celery ribs, carrot, onion, parsley, salt, and peppercorns. Add water to cover. Bring to boil over high heat, then lower heat and simmer for 20 minutes.

2. Remove chicken breasts from the saucepan. Cut meat into ½-inch cubes. Return to the saucepan and simmer to reduce stock.

3. In a skillet over medium heat, sauté butter, green peppers, chopped onion, celery, mushrooms, and rosemary until vegetables are soft. Add chicken, 1 cup chicken broth, and tomato sauce. Cook over medium heat until blended and hot.

4. Serve over spaghetti squash. Sprinkle with Parmesan cheese.

Home-Cooked Goodness

In this recipe, you cook the chicken to make chicken stock. Use any leftover stock as a base for soups and stews.

Chicken Verde

Yields 2 chickens and 3 cups sauce

Prep time: 15 minutes

Cook time: 1 hour

Serving size: 1/3 chicken (5 oz.) and 1/2 cup sauce

Each serving:

Glycemic index: low

Glycemic load: 1

Calories: 249

Protein: 38 grams

Carbohydrates: 4 grams

Fiber: 1 gram

Fat: 9 grams

Saturated fat: 4 grams

A mild-flavored stewed chicken with the comforting flavors of cilantro and tomatillos.

½ cup cilantro, chopped

2 cups onions, chopped

1 tsp. garlic, minced

1 (10-oz.) can tomatillas, drained with liquid reserved

½ tsp. salt

¼ tsp. freshly ground black pepper

2 TB. butter

2 (2.5-lb.) chickens, cut into serving pieces

1. Combine cilantro, onions, garlic, tomatillas, salt, and pepper in a food processor fitted with a chopping blade. Process until smooth. Add reserved tomatillo liquid and process until well blended.

2. In a large skillet over medium heat, heat butter and brown chicken pieces. Pour cilantro mixture over chicken and simmer, covered, about 1 hour, or until chicken is tender.

Tasty Tidbits

Spice up this mild Mexican chicken dish by adding a can of diced green chiles or a chopped jalapeño.

Turkey with Sausage and Vegetables

The mild flavor of turkey is enhanced with spicy sausages and fresh basil seasoning.

2 TB. butter

2 herb low-fat pork sausage links

1 lb. turkey breast, quartered

1 onion, finely sliced

3 carrots, coarsely chopped

4 tomatoes, chopped

1 TB. tomato paste

1 (15-oz.) can garbanzo beans

2 tsp. dried basil

1½ cups water

½ tsp. salt

¼ tsp. freshly ground black pepper

2 cups cooked basmati and wild rice

Yields 8 cups turkey mixture
Prep time: 20 minutes
Cook time: 1½ hours
Serving size: 1 cup
Each serving:
Glycemic index: low
Glycemic load: 13
Calories: 284
Protein: 22 grams
Carbohydrates: 31 grams
Fiber: 5 grams
Fat: 8 grams
Saturated fat: 3 grams

1. Heat butter in a saucepan. Sauté sausages until browned. Remove with a slotted spoon and drain on paper towels. Discard fat from the saucepan. Stir the turkey into the saucepan and cook until lightly browned.

2. Stir onion and carrot into the saucepan and brown lightly.

3. Add chopped tomatoes and tomato paste and simmer gently for about 5 minutes.

4. Chop sausage and return to the saucepan with beans, basil, water, salt, and pepper. Cover with a tight-fitting lid and cook gently for about 1 hour, until meat is tender.

5. Serve over basmati and wild rice.

Mediterranean Turkey Skewers

Enjoy the grilled taste of turkey and vegetables marinated in basil-and-garlic-flavored olive oil.

Yields 12 skewers
Prep time: 15 minutes, plus 30 minutes marinating time
Cook time: 10–15 minutes
Serving size: 3 skewers
Each serving:
Glycemic index: very low
Glycemic load: 0
Calories: 266
Protein: 21 grams
Carbohydrates: 5 grams
Fiber: 1 gram
Fat: 18 grams
Saturated fat: 5 grams

12 bamboo skewers

6 TB. olive oil

3 TB. lemon juice

1 tsp. garlic, minced

2 TB. fresh basil, chopped

½ tsp. salt

¼ tsp. freshly ground black pepper

1 (11-oz.) boned turkey, cut into 2-inch cubes

12–16 pickled onions

2 zucchini, cut into 1-inch slices

1 red or yellow bell pepper, cut into 2-inch squares

1. Soak bamboo skewers in water to prevent charring.

2. Mix olive oil with lemon juice, garlic, basil, salt, and pepper in a small bowl.

3. Prepare skewers by alternating turkey, onions, zucchini, and pepper pieces. Lay the prepared skewers on a platter and drizzle with olive oil mixture. Marinate for at least 30 minutes. Discard marinade.

4. Preheat the grill to medium high.

5. Grill skewers for 10 minutes, until vegetables are tender, turning occasionally. Serve hot.

Turkey Caesar Lasagna

Enjoy a new variation on Italian cuisine with this white Alfredo-style lasagna flavored with fresh basil.

9 dried whole-wheat lasagna noodles

1 recipe Cream Cheese Alfredo Sauce (see following recipe)

3 TB. lemon juice

½ tsp. freshly ground black pepper

3 cups shredded cooked turkey breast

1 (10-oz.) pkg. frozen chopped spinach, thawed and well drained

1 cup bottled roasted red sweet peppers, drained and chopped

2 cups fresh basil leaves

½ cup shredded Italian blend cheese

Yields 9 servings lasagna
Prep time: 35 minutes
Cook time: 50 minutes, plus 15 minutes stand time
Serving size: ¹/₉ recipe
Each serving:
Glycemic index: low
Glycemic load: 6
Calories: 152
Protein: 24 grams
Carbohydrates: 6 grams
Fiber: 2 grams
Fat: 3.57 grams
Saturated fat: 1.8 grams

1. Preheat the oven to 325°F.

2. Cook noodles until just before the al dente stage. Drain. Rinse with cold water; drain again. In a bowl, combine Alfredo sauce, lemon juice, and black pepper. Stir in turkey, spinach, and red peppers.

3. Arrange 3 noodles in bottom of 9×13-inch baking dish. Top with one third turkey mixture. Top with layer of fresh basil leaves. Repeat layers twice.

4. Cover and bake for 45–55 minutes or until heated through. Uncover. Sprinkle with cheese. Bake, uncovered, for 5 more minutes until cheese is melted. Let stand 15 minutes before serving.

Glycemic Notes

Use leftover turkey for this recipe, or use turkey breast from the deli. You can also bake a turkey breast for one dinner, and use the leftovers for this recipe. Substitute chicken if you prefer.

Alfredo Sauce with Cream Cheese

Yields 4 ½ cups sauce
Prep time: 10 minutes
Cook time: none
Serving size: ½ cup
Glycemic index: low
Glycemic load: 6
Calories: 235
Protein: 27 grams
Carbohydrates: 18 grams
Fiber: 2 grams
Fat: 22 grams
Saturated fat: 14 grams

½ cup butter

1 (8-oz.) package cream cheese

½ tsp. minced garlic

2 cups milk

¾ cup grated Parmesan cheese

⅛ tsp. ground black pepper

1. Melt butter in a medium-size saucepan over medium heat. Add cream cheese and garlic, stirring with a wire whisk until smooth.

2. Add milk, a little at a time, whisking to smooth out lumps. Stir in Parmesan and pepper. Remove from heat when sauce reaches desired consistency. Sauce will thicken rapidly—thin with milk if cooked too long.

3. Use with Turkey Caesar Lasagna, or serve over cooked vegetables, meats, or seafood pasta.

Variation: For lower fat, use olive oil in place of butter, low-fat cream cheese, skim milk and low-fat Parmesan cheese. Results: 205 calories, 19 grams fat, 6 grams saturated fat.

Home-Cooked Goodness

If you prefer a sauce lower in fat, substitute light cream cheese and low-fat milk.

Macadamia Turkey Steaks

Cook these when you have minimal time but want the maximum flavor found in macadamia-nut-crusted turkey steaks.

2 TB. whole-wheat flour	4 turkey breast steaks (4 oz. each)
1 egg, lightly beaten	
¾ cup macadamia nuts, finely chopped	2 TB. butter
	3 TB. olive oil
5 TB. grated Parmesan cheese	4 lemon wedges, to serve

1. Place flour on one plate, lightly beaten egg in a shallow bowl, and macadamia nuts mixed with Parmesan cheese on another plate.

2. Dip each side turkey steaks into flour and shake off any extra. Next, dip them into egg, and then gently press each side into nut and cheese mixture until evenly coated.

3. Heat butter and oil in a large frying pan and fry turkey steaks over medium heat for 2–3 minutes on each side, until golden. Garnish with fresh parsley sprigs and serve with lemon wedges.

Home-Cooked Goodness

This recipe calls for finely chopped macadamia nuts in lieu of high-glycemic breading. This gives you a more interesting flavor and a low-glycemic meal.

Yields 4 turkey breast steaks

Prep time: 15 minutes

Cook time: 10 minutes

Serving size: 1 turkey steak

Each serving:

Glycemic index: low

Glycemic load: 2

Calories: 459

Protein: 39 grams

Carbohydrates: 6 grams

Fiber: 1 gram

Fat: 31 grams

Saturated fat: 9 grams

Chapter 15

Seafood Main Dishes

In This Chapter

- ◆ Many fish and shellfish choices
- ◆ Purchasing fresh fish
- ◆ Adding flavor and pizzazz with sauces

Seafood can be a regular staple in your family menus when you eat based on the glycemic index. It offers great value—high levels of complete protein and good fats. Fish is zero on the glycemic index because it's a protein source with no carbohydrates. It's the sauces and recipe ingredients that add some carbohydrates.

Salmon au Poivre

Yields 4 salmon fillets
Prep time: 20 minutes
Cook time: 5 minutes
Serving size: 6 oz. lean salmon fillet
Each serving:
Glycemic index: low
Glycemic load: 2
Calories: 377
Protein: 42 grams
Carbohydrates: 5 grams
Fiber: <1 gram
Fat: 21 grams
Saturated fat: 3 grams

Rich salmon is flavored with the hot, peppery taste of coarsely ground black pepper and sweetened with a touch of honey.

4 (6-oz.) salmon fillets, skin removed

3 tsp. coarsely ground black pepper

2 TB. olive oil

½ cup natural chicken broth

1 TB. balsamic vinegar

1 TB. honey

¼ tsp. salt

1 (5- or 6-oz.) pkg. torn mixed salad greens

1 cup fresh strawberries, halved

2 TB. olive oil

1. Lightly coat each side of salmon with black pepper. In a large skillet over medium-high heat, heat olive oil. Add salmon fillets and cook for 1 minute in 2 tablespoons oil. Turn salmon over and slowly add chicken broth. Bring to boil, then reduce heat. Simmer, covered, for 5 minutes or until salmon flakes when tested with a fork.

2. While salmon simmers, whisk together remaining 2 tablespoons olive oil, balsamic vinegar, honey, and salt in a small bowl. Divide salad greens and strawberries among 4 individual serving plates. Drizzle greens with olive oil mixture.

3. Remove salmon from the skillet and place on greens.

Home-Cooked Goodness

Salmon is easy to prepare, and is especially healthy for your heart and beautifying for your skin with its concentration of omega-3 fatty acids.

Salmon with Red Cabbage

Salmon enhanced by the herbal flavors of garlic and basil, with the tang of fresh red cabbage slaw.

4 (5-oz.) fresh or frozen-and-thawed skinless salmon fillets

¼ cup balsamic vinegar

⅛ tsp. salt

¼ tsp. freshly ground black pepper

¼ cup prepared basil pesto

6 cups shredded red cabbage

2 green onions, bias-sliced

Yields 4 fillets and 4 cups cabbage
Prep time: 10 minutes
Cook time: 4–6 minutes per ½-inch thickness
Serving size: 1 fillet and 1 cup cabbage
Each serving:
Glycemic index: very low
Glycemic load: 0
Calories: 283
Protein: 38 grams
Carbohydrates: 8 grams
Fiber: 3 grams
Fat: 11 grams
Saturated fat: 1.7 grams

1. Preheat the broiler to high. Rinse salmon; pat dry with paper towels.

2. Place salmon on a rack of the broiler pan. Measure thickness of salmon. Brush each salmon fillet with 1 tablespoon vinegar. Sprinkle salmon with salt and pepper.

3. Broil salmon 4–5 inches from heat for 4–6 minutes per ½-inch thickness, or until salmon flakes easily with a fork.

4. In a bowl, whisk together remaining vinegar and pesto until combined. Set aside 2 tablespoons pesto mixture. Add cabbage to pesto mixture in the bowl; toss to coat.

5. To serve, divide cabbage mixture among 4 plates; top with salmon. Drizzle with reserved pesto mixture. Sprinkle with green onion slices.

Salmon with Avocado Salsa

Baked salmon is dressed with a creamy, spicy, chili-avocado sauce.

Yields 8 serving salmon with salsas
Prep time: 15 minutes
Bake time: 20 minutes
Serving size: 4-oz. salmon and ¼ cup avocado sauce
Each serving:
Glycemic index: very low
Glycemic load: 0
Calories: 305
Protein: 28 grams
Carbohydrates: 1 gram
Fiber: <1 gram
Fat: 21 grams
Saturated fat: 3 grams

1 (approx. 2 lbs.) salmon fillet

1 TB. butter

3 ripe avocados, peeled and seeded

¼ tsp. crushed red pepper

3 sprigs parsley

2 TB. green onions, chopped

¼ cup lemon juice

1 tsp. minced garlic

¼ tsp. salt

⅛ tsp. freshly ground black pepper

¼ cup fresh parsley, chopped

1 lemon, thinly sliced, for garnish

1. Preheat the oven to 375°F.

2. Place salmon flat, skin-side down, in a baking dish. Dot with butter. Place in the oven and bake 20 minutes. Remove salmon from the oven and transfer to a hot serving platter.

3. While salmon is baking, combine avocados, red pepper, parsley sprigs, green onions, lemon juice, garlic, salt, and pepper. Purée in an electric blender or a food processor fitted with a chopping blade, stirring down with a rubber spatula as necessary. When blended, spoon mixture over hot salmon. Sprinkle with parsley.

4. Garnish with lemon slices.

Home-Cooked Goodness

Shorten preparation time by dicing avocado and adding to ¼ cup all-natural salsa.

Salmon with Pumpkin Seed Pesto

The mild chili sauce imparts a warm, sunny flavor to the lime-infused salmon.

2 TB. olive oil

4 (5-oz.) salmon fillets

Juice of 1 lime, or 4 TB. fresh lime juice

2 tsp. dried lime rind

6 mild fresh red chiles

2 tsp. minced garlic

3 TB. pumpkin seeds

Juice of 1 lime, or 4 TB. fresh lime juice

2 tsp. dried lime rind

¼ salt

⅛ freshly ground black pepper

4 TB. olive oil

Yields 4 salmon fillets, plus ¾ cup sauce

Prep time: 20 minutes, plus 2 hours marinate time

Cook time: 10 minutes

Serving size: 1 fillet and 3 TB. sauce

Each serving:

Glycemic index: very low

Glycemic load: 0

Calories: 450

Protein: 36 grams

Carbohydrates: 1 gram

Fiber: <1 gram

Fat: 34 grams

Saturated fat: 3 grams

1. Rub olive oil into salmon. Place in a glass baking dish with a cover. Add first portion of lime juice and rind. Cover and marinate in the refrigerator for 2 hours, turning 2–3 times.

2. To make the chili sauce, seed chiles and place together with garlic, pumpkin seeds, second portion of lime juice, rind, salt, and pepper in a food processor fitted with a chopping blade. Process until well mixed. Pour in olive oil gradually over moving the blade until sauce has thickened.

3. Preheat the grill or broiler to medium-high.

4. Drain salmon from marinade. Grill or broil salmon 5 minutes per side and serve coated with chili sauce.

 Glycemic Notes _____

Overcooked salmon is hard and chewy and loses its flavor. Salmon is cooked when the flesh just turns opaque and can be flaked with a fork.

Salmon Croquettes

Yields 4 salmon patties
Prep time: 10 minutes
Cook time: 4 minutes
Serving size: 1 salmon patty
Each serving:
Glycemic index: low
Glycemic load: 2
Calories: 201
Protein: 12 grams
Carbohydrates: 5 grams
Fiber: <1 gram
Fat: 14 grams
Saturated fat: 2.2 grams

Quick-to-prepare salmon cakes flavored with zesty onion and parsley.

1 (6-oz.) pkg. salmon

2 eggs

1 small onion, finely chopped

2 tsp. dried parsley

½ tsp. salt

¼ tsp. pepper

¼ cup crushed stone-ground crackers

2 TB. olive oil

1. Drain salmon and place in a mixing bowl. Break into small pieces with a fork. Stir in eggs, onion, parsley, salt, pepper, and cracker crumbs.

2. Mix well and form into patties, using about ⅓ cup for each. In a skillet over medium-high heat, heat olive oil. Add salmon cakes and cook for 2 minutes per side. Drain on paper towels and serve.

Spice-Rubbed Halibut

Yields ¾ lb. halibut
Prep time: 10 minutes
Cook time: 8 minutes
Serving size: 3 oz. halibut
Each serving:
Glycemic index: very low
Glycemic load: 0
Calories: 102
Protein: 21 grams
Carbohydrates: 0 grams
Fiber: 0 grams
Fat: 2 grams
Saturated fat: <1 gram

Broiled halibut flavored with bold Indian spices of coriander, cumin, curry, and ginger.

¾ lb. halibut, cut into 1-inch-thick pieces

½ tsp. coriander

½ tsp. ground cumin

½ tsp. curry powder

¼ tsp. ground ginger

¼ tsp. salt

⅛ tsp. cayenne

1. Preheat the broiler to high.

2. Rinse fish and pat dry.

3. In a small bowl, mix coriander, cumin, curry powder, ginger, salt, and cayenne. Rub fish with spice mixture. Place pieces slightly apart in an 8-inch-square baking pan.

4. Broil 6 inches from heat for 3 minutes. With a wide spatula, turn fish over and broil until opaque, but still moist—about 3–5 minutes.

Tarragon Grilled Tuna

Tarragon imparts a fragrant mild, peppery taste that's accented with a lemon-based marinade.

4 (4-oz.) yellow-fin tuna steaks (1.5-inch thick)

2 TB. olive oil

2 tsp. finely chopped fresh tarragon, or 1 tsp. dried tarragon

½ tsp. salt

1 tsp. Dijon mustard

½ tsp. freshly ground black pepper

¼ cup fresh lemon juice

Yields 4 tuna steaks
Prep time: 5 minutes, plus 30 minutes refrigeration
Cook time: 8 minutes
Serving size: 1 tuna steak
Each serving:
Glycemic index: very low
Glycemic load: 0
Calories: 184
Protein: 28
Carbohydrates: 0 grams
Fiber: 0 grams
Fat: 8 grams
Saturated fat: 1 gram

1. Place tuna steaks in a large resealable plastic bag. Add oil, tarragon, salt, mustard, pepper, and lemon juice; seal bag. Turn bag to coat fish. Refrigerate at least 30 minutes.

2. When ready to cook, preheat the grill to medium. Remove tuna steaks from marinade and discard marinade. Place tuna on the grill. Cook 6–7 minutes, turning once, or until tuna is firm but still pink inside, and flakes easily with a fork.

Home-Cooked Goodness

You can also cook the tuna in your oven on high broil. Place tuna on the top layer of the broiling pan and cook as directed. Line the broiling pan with aluminum foil to make cleanup easy.

Tuna with Cannellini and Spinach

Cannellini beans and tuna enlivened with the flavors of oregano and garlic.

Yields 10 cups salad	
Prep time: 15 minutes	
Cook time: none	
Serving size: 1⅔ cup salad	
Each serving:	
Glycemic index: low	
Glycemic load: 5	
Calories: 139	
Protein: 13 grams	
Carbohydrates: 15 grams	
Fiber: 4 grams	
Fat: 3 grams	
Saturated fat: <1 gram	

2 (15-oz.) cans cannellini (white kidney) beans

1 TB. olive oil

1 tsp. minced garlic

½ tsp. dried oregano

¼ tsp. salt

⅛ tsp. freshly ground black pepper

1 cup celery, coarsely chopped, including some leaves

1 small red onion, sliced

1 (9-oz.) pkg. tuna, drained and separated into chunks

1–2 TB. fresh lemon juice

4 cups torn spinach leaves

1. Drain beans. In a mixing bowl, toss beans with olive oil, garlic, oregano, salt, and pepper. Add celery, onion, tuna, 3 tablespoons olive oil, and 2 tablespoons lemon juice. Toss well.

2. Arrange spinach leaves on a serving platter. Spoon beans mixture in center.

Tasty Tidbits

Canned legumes are a convenient way to obtain great flavor and taste while reducing preparation time. They're high in protein and fiber, and blend well with many different seasonings.

Pasta Shrimp with Broccoli and Cauliflower

Shrimp complements pasta flavored with traditional Italian accents of Parmesan, garlic, and parsley.

1 tsp. salt	**2 cups broccoli florets**
1 tsp. olive oil	**2 cups cauliflower florets**
1 cup dry whole-wheat pasta	**2 TB. olive oil**
1 TB. butter	**1 lb. peeled shrimp**
¼ cup Parmesan	**1 tsp. minced garlic**
¼ tsp. salt	**1 tsp. dried parsley**
¼ tsp. freshly ground black pepper	

1. Fill a large saucepan with water. Add salt and olive oil. Over high heat, bring to a boil. Add pasta and boil 5–6 minutes until not quite al dente. Drain. Toss with 2 tablespoons butter, Parmesan, salt, and pepper.

2. In a covered saucepan over high heat, lightly steam broccoli and cauliflower. Remove from heat.

3. While broccoli and cauliflower are steaming, heat olive oil in a small skillet over medium heat. Sauté shrimp with garlic and parsley.

4. To serve, toss pasta with shrimp, sauce from the pan, and vegetables.

Variation: For lower fat, use olive oil for butter and low-fat Parmesan cheese. Results: 392 calories, 12 grams fat, 2.3 grams saturated fat.

Yields 1 lb. shrimp, 4 cups vegetables, 4 cups pasta

Prep time: 10 minutes

Cook time: 20 minutes

Serving size: 1 cup pasta, 4 oz. shrimp, 1 cup vegetables

Each serving:
Glycemic index: very low
Glycemic load: 0
Calories: 405
Protein: 25 grams
Carbohydrates: 46 grams
Fiber: 9 grams
Fat: 13.5 grams
Saturated fat: 4.2 grams

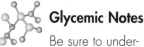

Glycemic Notes

Be sure to undercook pasta to keep it low glycemic.

Artichoke and Seafood Bake

Shrimp and crab baked with artichokes carry the European flavor of Swiss cheese, mushrooms, and dill.

Yields 12–15 cups bake
Prep time: 25 minutes
Cook time: 25 minutes
Serving size: 1½ cups bake
Each serving:
Glycemic index: very low
Glycemic load: 0
Calories: 221
Protein: 27 grams
Carbohydrates: 8 grams
Fiber: 2 grams
Fat: 9 grams
Saturated fat: 5 grams

4 TB. butter

2 TB. green onions, chopped

1 tsp. garlic, minced

½ lb. mushrooms, sliced

¼ cup flour

1 cup milk

⅔ cup dry white wine, fish stock, or clam juice

1½ cups Swiss cheese, grated

½ tsp. salt

¼ tsp. freshly ground black pepper

1 tsp. dried dill

1 lb. shrimp, cooked, shelled, and deveined

1 lb. lump crabmeat

1 pkg. frozen artichoke hearts, cooked and drained

1. Preheat the oven to 375°F.

2. Melt butter in a large skillet over medium-high heat, and sauté green onions with garlic until tender. Add mushrooms and cook 2 minutes.

3. Sprinkle mixture with flour, stir, and cook 1 minute.

4. Gradually stir in milk and wine, stock, or clam juices. Bring to boil, stirring until thick. Remove from heat and stir in 1 cup cheese until it melts. Stir in salt, pepper, and dill.

5. Add shrimp, crabmeat, and artichoke hearts and stir. Pour into a buttered baking dish. Sprinkle with remaining cheese.

6. Bake 25 minutes, or until bubbly.

Home-Cooked Goodness

This is a perfect dish for potlucks and buffet parties. Serve any leftovers as a special treat for breakfast or lunch.

Pacific Fish Stew

Tender pieces of seafood and fish flavored with tomato and rosemary create a hearty, aromatic stew.

3 TB. olive oil

1 onion, finely chopped

1 tsp. garlic, minced

½ cup fresh parsley, chopped

1 (28-oz.) can Italian plum tomatoes

2 (6-oz.) cans tomato paste

¼ tsp. rosemary, crushed

1 tsp. salt

½ tsp. freshly ground black pepper

2 cracked crabs

12 shucked clams with liquor

½ lb. shrimp, shelled and deveined

¾ lb. halibut fillet, cut into 4 pieces

Yields about 12 cups stew
Prep time: 15 minutes
Cook time: 2 hours 15 minutes
Serving size: 2 cups stew
Each serving:
Glycemic index: low
Glycemic load: 5
Calories: 312
Protein: 43 grams
Carbohydrates: 17 grams
Fiber: 3 grams
Fat: 8 grams
Saturated fat: 1 gram

Heat olive oil in a large saucepan over medium heat. Sauté onion and garlic until tender. Add parsley, tomatoes, tomato paste, rosemary, salt, and pepper. Bring to boil and simmer 2 hours, adding water if necessary. Add crabs, clams, shrimp, and halibut to sauce. Simmer 15 minutes, or until fish flakes easily.

Tuna and Corn Burgers

Fresh parsley flavor these broiled tuna burgers.

1½ cups mashed red potatoes

1 (7-oz.) pkg. tuna fish

¼ cup canned corn

2 TB. fresh parsley, chopped

¼ tsp. salt

⅛ tsp. freshly ground black pepper

⅛ cup coarse cornmeal

4 lemon wedges

Yields 8 burgers
Prep time: 10 minutes
Cook time: 6–10 minutes
Serving size: 2 burgers
Each serving:
Glycemic index: low
Glycemic load: 8
Calories: 116
Protein: 14 grams
Carbohydrates: 15 grams
Fiber: 1 gram
Fat: <1 gram
Saturated fat: 0 gram

1. Preheat the broiler to medium.

2. Place mashed potatoes in a mixing bowl. Stir in tuna, corn, chopped parsley, salt, and pepper. Shape into 8 patties. Place tuna cakes on a baking sheet sprinkled with coarse cornmeal.

3. Cook under a medium broiler until crisp and golden, about 6–10 minutes, turning once. Serve hot with lemon wedges.

Red Snapper in Butter Sauce

Yields 6 servings red snapper
Prep time: 10 minutes
Cook time: 30 minutes
Serving size: 4 oz. fish
Each serving:
Glycemic index: very low
Glycemic load: 0
Calories: 272
Protein: 32 grams
Carbohydrates: 0 grams
Fiber: 0 grams
Fat: 7.6 grams
Saturated fat: 4.8 grams

Tasty Tidbits

The unusual two-part cooking steps for the fish impart a satisfying buttery taste. Dressed with fresh lemon, this dish is elegant and memorable.

The preparation techniques intensify the rich, buttery flavor of the fish.

1 lemon	**¼ cup butter**
1 (1.5-lb.) red snapper	**2 TB. capers**
Salt and freshly ground black pepper	

1. Preheat the oven to 425°F.

2. Peel lemon, removing all white pulp. Cut lemon into thin slices and remove seeds. Cut each slice into small cubes, discarding membranes between sections. Reserve lemon cubes.

3. Rinse fish under cold water and pat dry with paper towels. Sprinkle fish inside and outside with salt and pepper.

4. Melt butter in a large oven-proof skillet over medium-high heat. When skillet is hot, add fish and cook only on one side for about 5 minutes. Tilt pan occasionally and spoon butter over fish.

5. Place fish in the oven and bake for about 25 minutes, or until fish flakes easily when tested with a fork.

6. Remove fish from the oven and transfer to a serving platter. Sprinkle with capers, reserved lemon cubes, and butter from the skillet.

Variation: Substitute striped bass and other small fish for the red snapper.

Mediterranean Cod and Asparagus

Olive tapenade flavors the cod with a tangy and earthy taste.

2 TB. plus 2 tsp. olive oil

6 (1.5-lbs.) cod fillets, skinned

¼ tsp. salt

⅛ tsp. freshly ground black pepper

1 lb. fresh asparagus spears, trimmed

6 TB. Olive Tapenade Relish—see Appetizer Chapter 8

Yields 6 cod fillets
Prep time: 15 minutes
Cook time: 12 minutes
Serving size: 1 cod fillet and 1½ TB. tapenade
Each serving:
Glycemic index: very low
Glycemic load: 0
Calories: 314
Protein: 44 grams
Carbohydrates: 3 grams
Fiber: 1 gram
Fat: 14 grams
Saturated fat: 1 gram

1. Preheat the oven to 475°F.

2. Lightly coat a large baking pan with 2 tablespoons olive oil. Arrange cod fillets on one side of the pan, turning under any thin portions. Brush fish with 1 teaspoon olive oil. Sprinkle with salt and black pepper.

3. Bake for 5 minutes. Place asparagus in opposite side of the pan. Brush with 1 teaspoon olive oil.

4. Bake 7–10 minutes more, or until cod flakes easily when tested with a fork. Serve fish with Olive Tapenade Relish and asparagus.

Home-Cooked Goodness

To save a cleanup step, line the baking dish with aluminum foil.

Cajun Catfish

Yields 4 catfish fillets and 1 cup vegetables
Prep time: 10 minutes
Cook time: 10 minutes
Serving size: 1 catfish fillet and ¼ cup vegetables
Each serving:
Glycemic index: very low
Glycemic load: 0
Calories: 256
Protein: 27 grams
Carbohydrates: 1 gram
Fiber: <1 gram
Fat: 16 grams
Saturated fat: 8.5 grams

Catfish flavored with spicy, hot Cajun spices and served with sautéed bell peppers.

1 tsp. dried thyme

1 tsp. dried oregano

1 tsp. freshly ground black pepper

¼ tsp. cayenne

2 tsp. paprika

½ tsp. garlic salt

4 (about 6 oz.) pieces lean, wild catfish

4 TB. butter

½ cup coarsely chopped red bell pepper

½ cup coarsely chopped green bell pepper

1. Place thyme, oregano, pepper, cayenne, paprika, and garlic salt in a bowl and mix well. Dip fish fillets in spice mixture to coat lightly.

2. Heat 2 tablespoons butter in a large skillet over medium heat. Add peppers, and sauté for 4–5 minutes, until softened. Remove peppers to a side plate.

3. Add remaining butter to the skillet and increase to medium-high heat. Add catfish fillets and cook for about 3–4 minutes per side, until browned and cooked.

4. Transfer fish to a serving platter, and surround with peppers.

Home-Cooked Goodness

When frying or sautéing, it's great to use a kitchen utensil called a spatter screen. Place over the top of your pan and it catches oil spatters, preventing them from landing on your cooktop and kitchen counters. Available where kitchen utensils are sold.

Crab Cakes

Crab cakes are lightly flavored with mustard and cayenne to bring out the rich crab taste.

½ cup mayonnaise

2 tsp. dry mustard

Pinch of salt

Pinch of cayenne

1 celery stalk, finely minced

2 green onions, finely minced

1 lb. cooked crabmeat

1 cups fresh sourdough bread crumbs

4 tsp. butter

4 tsp. olive oil

4 lemon wedges

Yields 8 patties
Prep time: 15 minutes
Cook time: 7 minutes
Serving size: 1 patty
Each serving:
Glycemic index: low
Glycemic load: 3
Calories: 199
Protein: 13 grams
Carbohydrates: 4 grams
Fiber: <1 gram
Fat: 15 grams
Saturated fat: 3 grams

1. In a mixing bowl, stir together mayonnaise, mustard, salt, and cayenne. Stir in celery and green onions. Gently fold in crabmeat and half of bread crumbs.

2. Shape crab mixture into 8 patties, each 1-inch thick. (They won't hold together well.)

3. Heat 2 large frying pans over medium heat. In each pan, melt 2 teaspoons butter with 2 teaspoons oil. Place 4 crab cakes in each pan and cook until golden brown, about 3 minutes. Turn and cook 3–4 minutes longer, until cakes are well browned on second side and hot throughout.

4. Transfer to individual plates and serve at once with lemon wedges.

Scallops with Bacon

Scallops are given extra flavor with crisp bacon.

Yields 1½ lbs. scallops
Prep time: 10 minutes, plus 30 minutes marinate time
Cook time: 8–10 minutes
Serving size: 4 oz. scallops, plus bacon wrapping
Each serving:
Glycemic index: very low
Glycemic load: 0
Calories: 196
Protein: 31 grams
Carbohydrates: 0 grams
Fiber: 0 grams
Fat: 8 grams
Saturated fat: 1.6 grams

1½ lbs. sea scallops
4 TB. lemon juice
2 TB. olive oil

⅛ tsp. freshly ground black pepper
6– slices bacon, cut in half

1. Rinse scallops and blot dry with a clean kitchen towel. In a glass bowl, mix lemon juice, olive oil, and pepper. Add scallops and marinate in the refrigerator for at least 30 minutes.

2. Heat the oven broiler to high. Wrap each scallop with ½ strip bacon and secure with a toothpick.

3. Place scallops on the top level of the broiler pan. Broil until golden brown and bacon is crisp to your preference.

Baked Tilapia with Mango

Mango avocado sauce with fresh basil flavors this delicate fish.

Yields 4 fillets plus 1½ cups sauce
Prep time: 10 minutes
Cook time: 7–10 minutes
Serving size: 4–5 ounces fish and ⅓ cup sauce
Each serving:
Glycemic index: low
Glycemic load: 3
Calories: 294
Protein: 35 grams
Carbohydrates: 7 grams
Fiber: 1 gram
Fat: 14 grams
Saturated fat: 1 gram

1 TB. olive oil
4 tilapia fillets (4–5-oz. each)
¼ tsp. garlic powder
¼ tsp. dried basil
¼ tsp. dried marjoram

¼ tsp. salt
⅛ tsp. freshly ground black pepper
1 avocado, diced
1 cup mango, diced
2 TB. fresh basil, chopped

1. Preheat the oven to 350°F.

2. Brush olive oil on both sides of fish. Place fish in a shallow baking dish. Sprinkle with garlic powder, basil, marjoram, salt, and pepper.

3. In a small bowl, mix avocado, mango, and fresh basil. Bake 7–10 minutes until fish is opaque in center. Remove to a serving platter. Top with avocado mango mixture.

Grilled Clams with Tarragon Butter

The tarragon adds a sweet peppery taste to the clams.

36 small hard-shell clams, such as littlenecks (about 5 lbs.)

4 quarts water

⅓ cup salt

4 TB. butter

1 tsp. dried tarragon

2 TB. fresh lemon juice

Dash salt and pepper

Yields 36 clams
Prep time: 15 minutes
Cook time: 6–8 minutes
Serving size: 9 clams (4.5-oz.) and 1 TB. sauce
Each serving:
Glycemic index: very low
Glycemic load: 0
Calories: 236
Protein: 32 grams
Carbohydrates: 0 grams
Fiber: 0 grams
Fat: 12 grams
Saturated fat: 7.3 grams

1. Preheat the grill to medium high.

2. Scrub clams under cold running water. In a 6- to 8-quart stockpot, stir together 4 quarts water and ⅓ cup salt. Add clams. Soak for 15 minutes. Drain, discarding water. Rinse clams. Repeat twice.

3. In a small microwavable bowl, place butter, tarragon, lemon juice, and dash salt and pepper. Microwave on high 30 seconds until butter is melted. Remove from the microwave and stir.

4. Arrange clams in a single layer on a rack on the grill over medium-high for 6–8 minutes or until opened at least ½ inch, turning once. Remove clams as they open and keep warm while others cook. Discard unopened clams. Serve with tarragon butter.

Monkfish with Mexican Salsa

Salsa adds a tangy, zingy flavor to the monkfish.

Yields 4 monkfish pieces and 4 cups salsa
Prep time: 15 minutes, plus 30 minutes marinate time
Cook time: 6–8 minutes
Serving size: 5 oz. monk-fish and 1 cup salsa
Each serving:
Glycemic index: low
Glycemic load: 1
Calories: 379
Protein: 28 grams
Carbohydrates: 6 grams
Fiber: 1 gram
Fat: 27 grams
Saturated fat: 2 grams

4 tomatoes, seeded, peeled, and diced

1 avocado, pitted, peeled, and diced

½ red onion, chopped

1 green chili, seeded and chopped

2 TB. fresh cilantro, chopped

2 TB. olive oil

1 TB. lime juice

4 (5-oz.) pieces monkfish

3 TB. olive oil

2 TB. lime juice

1 tsp. minced garlic

1 TB. fresh cilantro, chopped

¼ tsp. salt

⅛ tsp. freshly ground black pepper

1. In a mixing bowl, add tomatoes, avocado, red onion, green chili, 2 tablespoons cilantro, olive oil, and lime juice. Mix ingredients. Let stand while you prepare and marinate fish.

2. Mix together oil, lime juice, garlic, 1 tablespoon cilantro, salt, and pepper in a shallow glass dish. Add monkfish and coat with marinade, turning several times. Cover dish and marinate in the refrigerator for 30 minutes.

3. Preheat the oven broiler to high.

4. Remove monkfish from marinade to the top of an oven broiling pan. Broil for 10–12 minutes, turning once and brushing regularly with marinade until cooked through.

5. Serve monkfish accompanied with salsa.

Tasty Tidbits

If you marinate fish longer than 15 minutes, do so in the refrigerator to preserve freshness and to hamper the growth of microorganisms.

Trout Baked in Foil

Trout takes on the delicate citrus flavors of lemon and orange.

4 trout

Salt and freshly ground black pepper

1 tsp. garlic powder

8 thin lemon slices

4 TB. dry white wine

4 TB. orange juice

4 TB. butter

Yields 4 fish
Prep time: 15 minutes
Cook time: 25 minutes
Serving size: 1 (4-oz.) fish
Each serving:
Glycemic index: low
Glycemic load: 1
Calories: 291
Protein: 28 grams
Carbohydrates: 2 grams
Fiber: 0 grams
Fat: 19 grams
Saturated fat: 8.75 grams

1. Preheat the oven to 350°F.

2. Place each fish on a piece of aluminum foil big enough to enclose it when folded as a package.

3. Sprinkle inside cavity of each fish with salt, pepper, and garlic. Place 2 lemon slices on top each fish. Sprinkle each with 1 tablespoon wine and 1 tablespoon orange juice. Dot each with 1 tablespoon butter. Fold up foil so that package is sealed.

4. Bake about 25 minutes, until fish flakes and is opaque in middle.

Chapter 16

Vegetarian Main Dishes

In This Chapter

- Satisfying vegetarian meals
- Keeping the glycemic value low
- Blending interesting flavors and vegetables

The challenge in eating vegetarian meals and eating low glycemic is to focus on eating vegetables and legumes and avoid the white and fluffy starches. Then add some low-glycemic breads, pastas, and rice to your meals, keeping in mind that they increase the glycemic load for the meal.

In this chapter we offer you interesting and varied recipes that include legumes, bean curd or tofu, and plenty of vegetables. You'll find many different flavors, too, such as curry, Italian, Mexican, and Southern. You'll enjoy new cuisine tastes of portabella mushroom burgers and tofu kabobs.

Keep a watchful eye on serving size and glycemic load in these recipes to ensure your glycemic eating success.

Broccoli and Chestnut Terrine

The sweetness of nutmeg gently flavors the terrine along with yogurt and Parmesan cheese.

Yields 1 loaf pan	

Prep time: 20 minutes

Cook time: 20–25 minutes

Serving size: 1 (1.5-inch) slice

Each serving:

Glycemic index: low

Glycemic load: 4

Calories: 109

Protein: 7 grams

Carbohydrates: 18 grams

Fiber: 3 grams

Fat: 1 gram

Saturated fat: 4 grams

4 cups broccoli florets

2 cups cooked water chestnuts, coarsely chopped

½ cup fresh stone-ground bread crumbs

½ cup oat bran

4 TB. low-fat plain yogurt

2 TB. finely shredded Parmesan cheese

½ tsp. salt

⅛ tsp. nutmeg

¼ tsp. freshly ground black pepper

3 eggs, beaten

1. Preheat the oven to 350°F. Line a 9×5×3-inch loaf pan with nonstick baking parchment.

2. Blanch or steam broccoli for 3–4 minutes until just tender. Drain well. Reserve a quarter of the smallest florets and finely chop the rest.

3. Mix chestnuts, bread crumbs, oat bran yogurt, and Parmesan. Stir in salt, nutmeg, and pepper. Fold in chopped broccoli, reserved florets, and beaten eggs.

4. Spoon broccoli mixture into a prepared pan.

5. Place the loaf pan in a roasting pan and pour boiling water to come halfway up sides of the loaf pan. Bake for 20–25 minutes. Remove from the oven. Turn out onto a plate or tray.

Home-Cooked Goodness

Make your own bread crumbs in the food processor fitted with the chopping blade. Tear bread into bite-size pieces and process for 30 to 60 seconds.

Super Nachos

Nachos flavored with freshly sautéed onions, green chiles, and taco sauce.

2 TB. olive oil

1 large onion, chopped

1 (29-oz.) can no fat added refried beans

1 (4.5-oz.) can chopped green chiles

2 cups grated low-fat Monterey Jack cheese

¾ cup green taco sauce

1 cup light dairy sour cream

1 cup chopped green onion

1 cup chopped black olives

2 cups sliced jicama

2 cups sliced zucchini

2 cups sliced carrots

Yields 10 cups nachos plus 6 cups vegetables
Prep time: 15 minutes
Cook time: 20 minutes
Serving size: 1 cup nachos plus ⅔ cup vegetables
Each serving:
Glycemic index: low
Glycemic load: 5
Calories: 198
Protein: 10 grams
Carbohydrates: 17 grams
Fiber: 6 grams
Fat: 10 grams
Saturated fat: 2.81 grams

1. Preheat the oven to 400°F.

2. In a skillet over medium-high heat, heat olive oil and add onions. Sauté onions until they turn translucent but not browned.

3. In a shallow 9×13-inch glass baking pan, spread beans evenly. Top with sautéed onions, chiles, and grated cheese. Drizzle green taco sauce over all.

4. Bake at 400°F for 15 minutes. Remove from the oven. Cover with dairy sour cream. Sprinkle green onions over sour cream and top with chopped olives. Return to the oven for 5 minutes.

5. Serve with jicama, zucchini, and carrots for dipping.

 Glycemic Notes

By using sliced vegetables as dippers, you keep the glycemic value of nachos in the low category. If you ate traditional corn chips, your meal would move into the medium-to-high range.

Vegetable Lasagna

Yields 1 (9×13-inch) pan lasagna
Prep time: 25 minutes
Cook time: 1 hour, plus 20 minutes stand time
Serving size: 1 square, about 3×4 inches
Each serving:
Glycemic index: low
Glycemic load: 17
Calories: 475
Protein: 37 grams
Carbohydrates: 39 grams
Fiber: 6 grams
Fat: 19 grams
Saturated fat: 11 grams

Vegetables and noodles flavored with oregano and basil topped with Italian cheeses.

1 lb. lasagna noodles	1 tsp. dried oregano
1½ TB. olive oil	1 tsp. dried basil
2 green peppers, chopped	¼ tsp. black pepper
2 large onions, chopped	2 lbs. Ricotta cheese
¾ lb. sliced mushrooms	1 lb. Mozzarella cheese, grated
5 carrots, grated	
4 cups diced tomatoes	¾ cup grated Parmesan cheese
1 (1-lb. 10-oz.) jar pasta sauce	

1. Cook lasagna noodles per package instructions. Cook not quite to al dente. Remove from heat, drain, and rinse.

2. Preheat the oven to 350°F.

3. In a large skillet over medium heat, heat oil and sauté peppers, onions, mushrooms, and carrots until tender. Add tomatoes, sauce, and spices. Simmer 10–15 minutes.

4. In a shallow 9×13 glass baking dish, place ⅓ tomato mixture. Cover with ⅓ noodles. Spread ⅓ Ricotta cheese on noodles and sprinkle with ⅓ Mozzarella.

5. Continue layering with tomato mixture, noodles, Ricotta cheese, and Mozzarella until they're all used. Top lasagna with Parmesan.

6. Bake 1 hour at 350°F until hot and bubbly. Remove from the oven. Let stand 20 minutes before cutting.

Variation: For lower fat, use low-fat versions of ricotta, Mozzarella, and Parmesan cheese. Results: 271 calories, 9 grams fat, 4 grams saturated fat.

Tasty Tidbits

Let the lasagna stand uncut for 20–30 minutes upon removing from the oven. This lets it settle and solidify enough for you to cut without it being runny.

Bean, Carrot, and Cabbage Salad

The salad is flavored with onion and sweet pickle relish.

1 (15-oz.) can pinto beans, drained

½ cup coarsely shredded carrot

½ cup shredded cabbage

1 small onion, grated

¼ cup sweet pickle relish

½ tsp. salt

¼ tsp. freshly ground black pepper

⅓ cup Italian salad dressing

4 lettuce leaves

Yields 4 cups salad
Prep time: 10 minutes
Cook time: none
Serving size: 1 cup salad
Each serving:
Glycemic index: low
Glycemic load: 7
Calories: 208
Protein: 7 grams
Carbohydrates: 23 grams
Fiber: 6 grams
Fat: 6 grams
Saturated fat: 1 gram

1. In a salad bowl, combine pinto beans, carrot, cabbage, onion, relish, salt, pepper, and dressing. Toss to blend.

2. On individual plates, serve on lettuce leaves.

Variation: Substitute black beans or kidney beans for the pinto

Home-Cooked Goodness

Our recipes call for canned legumes for convenience and ease of preparation. If you prefer home-cooked legumes, you can soak the beans the night before, and cook up a batch the next day before preparing your recipe.

Bean Curd and Crunchy Vegetables

A stir-fry seasoned with sesame oil and flavored with soy sauce.

Yields 9 cups, plus 2 cups rice
Prep time: 15 minutes, plus 30 minutes marinate time
Cook time: 10 minutes
Serving size: 1½ cups bean curd and vegetables with ⅓ cup rice
Each serving:
Glycemic index: low
Glycemic load: 11
Calories: 374
Protein: 22 grams
Carbohydrates: 39 grams
Fiber: 12 grams
Fat: 14.5 grams
Saturated fat: 1.5 grams

2 (8-oz.) packages smoked bean curd, cut into ½-inch cubes

3 TB. soy sauce

2 TB. dry sherry or vermouth

1 TB. sesame oil

3 TB. olive oil

2 green onions, thinly sliced

2 carrots, cut into sticks

1 cup small broccoli florets

1 large zucchini, thinly sliced

4 oz. baby corn, halved

4 oz. button or shiitake mushrooms, sliced

1 TB. sesame seeds

2 cups basmati rice, cooked

1. Marinate bean curd in soy sauce, sherry or vermouth, and sesame oil for at least 30 minutes. Drain and reserve marinade.

2. Heat olive oil in a wok over medium-high heat. Stir-fry bean curd until browned. Remove to a side plate.

3. Stir-fry green onions, carrots, broccoli, zucchini, and baby corn, stirring and tossing for about 2 minutes. Add mushrooms and cook 1 minute.

4. Return bean curd to the wok and pour in marinade. Heat to boiling. Remove from heat and sprinkle with sesame seeds.

5. Serve immediately with rice.

Corn and Bean Tamale Pie

A rich tamale pie topped with polenta and flavored with oregano, cumin, and garlic.

1 onion, chopped

2 tsp. minced garlic

1 red bell pepper, seeded and chopped

2 TB. oil

2 green chiles, seeded and chopped

2 TB. ground cumin

1 lb. ripe tomatoes, peeled, seeded, and chopped

1 TB. tomato paste

1 (15-oz.) can red kidney beans, drained and rinsed

1 (10-oz.) pkg. whole-kernel corn

1 TB. chopped fresh oregano

½ tsp. salt

¼ tsp. freshly ground black pepper

1 cup uncooked coarse polenta

1 TB. flour

½ tsp. salt

2 tsp. baking powder

1 egg, lightly beaten

½ cup 2 percent milk,

1 TB. butter, melted

½ cup grated smoked cheddar cheese

Yields 1 (9×13-inch) pie		
Prep time: 20 minutes		
Cook time: 40 minutes		
Serving size: 1 (3×4-inch) serving		
Each serving:		
Glycemic index: low		
Glycemic load: 4		
Calories: 127		
Protein: 5 grams		
Carbohydrates: 16 grams		
Fiber: 3 grams		
Fat: 5.26 grams		
Saturated fat: 2.16 grams		

1. Preheat the oven to 425°F.

2. In a skillet over medium-high heat, sauté onion, garlic, and pepper in olive oil for 5 minutes, until softened. Add chiles and cumin; sauté for 1 minute. Stir in tomatoes, tomato paste, beans, corn kernels, and oregano. Add salt and pepper. Simmer, uncovered, for 10 minutes.

3. To make topping, mix polenta, flour, salt, baking powder, egg, milk, and butter to form a thick batter.

4. Transfer bean mixture to a 9×13-inch glass baking dish. Spoon polenta mixture over and spread evenly.

5. Bake for 30 minutes. Remove from the oven. Sprinkle with cheese. Bake for 5–10 minutes, until golden.

 Tasty Tidbits

You can prepare the pie ahead of time and store in the refrigerator until it's time to bake. Bring to room temperature before baking, or add 5–10 minutes to the baking time.

Lentil Sauté

Artichokes, mushrooms, and snow peas in a light cream sauce flavored with onion and topped with almonds.

1 cup snow peas	**4 TB. light cream**
2 TB. butter	**¼ cup slivered almonds, toasted**
1 small onion, chopped	
1 cup mushrooms, sliced	**½ tsp. salt**
1 (14-oz.) can artichoke hearts, drained and halved	**¼ tsp. freshly ground black pepper**
1 (14-oz.) can green lentils, drained	

Yields 6 cups lentils

Prep time: 10 minutes

Cook time: 15 minutes

Serving size: 1½ cup sauté

Each serving:

Glycemic index: low

Glycemic load: 4

Calories: 236

Protein: 7 grams

Carbohydrates: 21 grams

Fiber: 5 grams

Fat: 13.8 grams

Saturated fat: 6.65 grams

1. Bring a saucepan of salted water to boil over high heat. Add snow peas, and cook for 4 minutes until just tender. Drain. Rinse snow peas under cold water. Drain. Pat dry with paper towels and set aside.

2. Melt butter in a large skillet over medium heat and sauté onion for 2–3 minutes.

3. Add sliced mushrooms. Sauté for 2–3 minutes. Add artichoke hearts, snow peas, and lentils. Sauté for 2 minutes.

4. Stir in cream and almonds. Cook for 1 minute. Stir in salt and black pepper.

Mushroom Burgers

Portabella mushrooms lend substantial texture and flavor coupled with Italian dressing and grilled onions.

4 large portabella mushroom caps, about 3 oz. each

1 large red pepper, quartered and cored

3 TB. Italian salad dressing

3 TB. mayonnaise

4 small stone-ground whole-wheat dinner rolls, cut in half like hamburger buns

4 lettuce leaves

4 thick slices tomato

1½ cups thickly sliced red onion

Yields 4 burgers
Prep time: 10 minutes
Cook time: 12 minutes
Serving size: 1 burger
Each serving:
Glycemic index: low
Glycemic load: 9
Calories: 242
Protein: 8 grams
Carbohydrates: 27 grams
Fiber: 4 grams
Fat: 11.3 grams
Saturated fat: 1.3 grams

1. Heat the grill to medium-high.

2. Grill onion slices 4 minutes on a side. Grill mushrooms and peppers 5–6 minutes on a side. Cook until vegetables are lightly browned.

3. Whisk salad dressing and mayonnaise in a small bowl. Spread on buns.

4. On bottom half of bun layer, put lettuce, tomato, mushroom cap, piece red pepper, and ¼ onions. Cover with top of bun. Serve.

Home-Cooked Goodness

Use a special grill accessory to hold small or fragile items such as vegetables or fish. It prevents them from falling through the grill into the coals.

Black Bean Chili

Chili accented with mole flavor topped with sour cream and cilantro.

Yields 8 cups, plus 2 cups rice
Prep time: 10 minutes
Cook time: 15 minutes
Serving size: 1¹/₃ cup chili and ¹/₃ cup rice
Each serving:
Glycemic index: low
Glycemic load: 17
Calories: 200
Protein: 8 grams
Carbohydrates: 38 grams
Fiber: 8 grams
Fat: 1.68 grams
Saturated fat: 1 gram

2 (10-oz.) can diced tomatoes and green chiles

1 (19-oz.) can black beans, drained

1 (10-oz.) box frozen corn

¼ cup tomato paste

4 TB. fresh lime juice

½ tsp. bitter cocoa powder

¼ tsp. chili powder

2 cups cooked brown rice

¼ cup sour cream

¼ cup chopped fresh cilantro

1. In large saucepan over medium-high heat, stir together tomatoes and green chiles, black beans, corn, tomato paste, lime juice, cocoa powder, and chili powder. Cook, stirring occasionally for 10 minutes or until thoroughly heated.

2. Serve over rice topped with sour cream and chopped cilantro.

Eggplant Parmesan

A layered pie flavored with oregano and marinara sauce.

2 eggplants, cut in ½-inch-thick rounds

¼ cup olive oil

1 tsp. salt

½ tsp. freshly ground black pepper

1 (20-oz.) jar marinara sauce

1 tsp. oregano

1½ cups shredded Mozzarella (part skim milk) cheese

1 cup shaved Parmesan cheese

Yields 1 (9×9-inch) pan
Prep time: 20 minutes
Cook time: 53 minutes plus 45 minutes stand time
Serving size: 1 (4.5×1.5-inch) square
Each serving:
Glycemic index: low
Glycemic load: 4
Calories: 280
Protein: 13 grams
Carbohydrates: 21 grams
Fiber: 7 grams
Fat: 16 grams
Saturated fat: 4.31 grams

1. Heat the oven broiler to high.

2. Place half of eggplant rounds on top of the broiler pan. Brush lightly with olive oil and sprinkle with salt and pepper. Broil 6–8 minutes per side. Remove eggplant rounds and repeat with other half of rounds.

3. Preheat the oven to 350°F.

4. In a 9×9-inch shallow glass baking dish, spread ½ cup marinara sauce. Top with half of eggplant rounds. Spoon on 1¼ cup sauce. Sprinkle with ½ teaspoon oregano, top with 1 cup mozzarella, ½ cup Parmesan, rest of eggplant, sauce, oregano, and mozzarella. Sprinkle with remaining Parmesan. Cover with foil.

5. Bake for 45 minutes or until bubbly. Let stand 15 minutes before serving.

Variation: For lower fat, use lite mozzarella (2.5 g fat/oz.) and low-fat Parmesan. Results: 141 calories, 5 grams fat, 3 grams saturated fat.

Tasty Tidbits

Increase the protein value of this recipe by adding 4 ounces of crumbled or sliced tofu between layers.

Tofu and Bell Pepper Kabobs

Kabobs accented with salted peanuts and dipped in sweet chili sauce.

Yields 8–12 kabobs
Prep time: 15 minutes
Cook time: 10 minutes
Serving size: 2 oz. tofu, 1 bell pepper
Each serving:
Glycemic index: very low
Glycemic load: 1
Calories: 255
Protein: 17 grams
Carbohydrates: 13 grams
Fiber: 6 grams
Fat: 15.5 grams
Saturated fat: 2.17 grams

9 ounces firm tofu, drained

½ cup finely chopped salted peanuts

2 red bell peppers, seeded, cored, and cut into 1¼-inch squares

2 green bell peppers, seeded, cored, and cut into 1¼-inch squares

8–12 bamboo skewers, soaked in water

4 TB. Thai sweet chili dipping sauce

1. Heat the broiler to medium.

2. Cut tofu into 1-inch cubes. Place peanuts on a side plate. Press tofu cubes into peanuts to coat.

3. Prepare kabobs by alternating tofu with pepper squares on bamboo skewers.

4. Place kabobs on the top level of the oven broiler pan. Broil for 10–12 minutes until peppers and peanuts begin to brown.

5. Serve kabobs with dipping sauce.

Tasty Tidbits

Serve these kabobs as a main course, or for an appetizer. They're easy to eat and would be delicious with sesame seeds or cashews in place of the peanuts.

Red Beans and Rice

A traditional classic dish flavored with hot pepper sauce, garlic, and thyme.

1 cup Uncle Ben's converted rice, cooked per package directions

1 TB. olive oil

2 stalks celery with leaves

1 medium red onion, coarsely chopped

2 tsp. minced garlic

½ tsp. dried thyme

1 bay leaf

2 (15–19-oz.) cans red kidney beans, rinsed and drained

1 cup water

¼ cup fresh chopped parsley

1 tsp. Worcestershire sauce

⅛ tsp. hot pepper sauce

Yields 8 cups, plus 2 cups rice
Prep time: 10 minutes
Cook time: 20 minutes
Serving size: 1 cup beans with ¼ cup rice
Each serving:
Glycemic index: low
Glycemic load: 7
Calories: 238
Protein: 7 grams
Carbohydrates: 24 grams
Fiber: 7 grams
Fat: 2 grams
Saturated fat: <1 gram

1. Prepare rice per package directions.

2. In a large saucepan over medium heat, heat oil. Sauté celery, onion, garlic, thyme, and bay leaf. Cook until vegetables are tender, about 10 minutes.

3. Stir in beans, water, parsley, Worcestershire, and hot pepper sauce. Cook until heated. Discard bay leaf.

4. To serve, spoon rice into bowls. Top with bean mixture.

Home-Cooked Goodness

Uncle Ben's Converted Rice is low glycemic even though it's not nutrient-dense. You can also use brown rice for a crunchier texture and more nutritional value.

Garbanzo Bean and Sweet Potato Stew

Yields 10 cups stew
Prep time: 15 minutes
Cook time: 20 minutes
Serving size: 1¼ cup stew
Each serving:
Glycemic index: low
Glycemic load: 16
Calories: 204
Protein: 7 grams
Carbohydrates: 35 grams
Fiber: 4 grams
Fat: 4 grams
Saturated fat: <1 gram

A satisfying vegetable stew flavored with coriander and curry.

2 TB. olive oil

1 cup chopped onion

1 green pepper, diced

1 TB. minced garlic

1 tsp. coriander

1 tsp. curry powder

1 (28-oz.) can whole tomatoes, chopped

4 cups sweet coarsely diced sweet potatoes

1 (19-oz.) can garbanzo beans

1 tsp. salt

¼ tsp. freshly ground black pepper

½ cup fresh cilantro

1. In a large skillet over medium heat, heat oil and sauté onion, pepper, and garlic. Cook about 6 minutes, until vegetables are tender.

2. Stir in coriander, curry powder, tomatoes, sweet potatoes, garbanzo beans, salt, and pepper. Bring to a boil. Reduce heat, cover and simmer 10–15 minutes, stirring once or twice until sweet potatoes are tender. Stir in cilantro.

Glycemic Notes

Serve this stew with a green salad to keep the glycemic load low. If you served it with bread or crackers, the total glycemic load could be too high for the meal.

Part 5

On the Side

With so many varied salad, vegetable, and fruit side dishes to choose from, you'll find it easy to eat the recommended 2-3 per meal.

Yes, you can eat potatoes. Our recipes give you choices for roasting, casseroles, and potato salads. The grains chapter gives you many ways to cook savory pilafs, polenta, and others for crunchy low-glycemic starches.

Chapter 17

Side Salads

In This Chapter

- ◆ Dressing up your meals
- ◆ High-level nutrition in colorful servings
- ◆ Quick homemade dressings

The salads we created for you are luxurious farm-sourced gems packed with high-level nutrition. They're beautiful—colorful, aromatic, and the combination of ingredients and dressings make them irresistible.

Always purchase the freshest and crispest salad vegetables you can find. If the produce on the shelves looks tired, ask the produce department staff to bring out fresher choices.

Homemade salad dressings are simple when you know the basics. Salad dressings have two main ingredients: oil and vinegar or lemon juice in the approximate ratio of 3:1. For $^3/_4$ cup oil, you'd use $^1/_4$ cup vinegar or lemon juice.

Then add in seasonings, mustards, grated cheeses, and other savory or sweet ingredients to add sparkle to your salad fixings. Keep these items on hand in your kitchen for salad dressings.

Wild Rice Salad with Artichokes

Yields 10 cups salad
Prep time: 15 minutes
Cook time: 45 minutes
Serving size: 1 cup salad
Each serving (salad):
Glycemic index: low
Glycemic load: 7
Calories: 134
Protein: 8 grams
Carbohydrates: 21 grams
Fiber: 5.5 grams
Fat: 2 grams
Saturated fat: <1 gram
Each serving (salad dressing per TB.):
Glycemic index: very low
Glycemic load: 0
Calories: 108
Protein: 0 grams
Carbohydrates: 0 grams
Fiber: 0 grams
Fat: 12 grams
Saturated fat: <1 gram

The nutty taste of wild rice and cheese enhances the flavor of artichokes and peas.

1 cup olive oil

⅓ cup white wine vinegar

¼ tsp. salt

1 tsp. celery seed

½ tsp. freshly ground black pepper

¼ tsp. dry mustard

¼ tsp. paprika

1 tsp. minced garlic

2 quarts plus 1 cup water

3 cups wild rice

1 (14-oz.) can artichoke hearts

1 (10-oz.) pkg. frozen peas

1 green bell pepper, chopped

1 bunch green onions, chopped

1 pint cherry tomatoes, halved

2 TB. toasted slivered almonds

¼ cup shredded Parmesan cheese

1. To make dressing, combine olive oil, vinegar, salt, celery seed, pepper, mustard, paprika, and garlic in a lidded jar. Shake well. Refrigerate until ready to use.

2. In a large saucepan over high heat, bring water and rice to boil. Reduce heat to low, cover and simmer for 30 minutes. Drain rice.

3. Drain artichoke hearts. Place in a salad bowl. Halve artichoke hearts and add to rice with peas, green pepper, green onions, and tomatoes. Toss with desired amount of dressing.

4. Sprinkle with almonds and Parmesan cheese. Serve with salad tongs or a slotted spoon.

Tasty Tidbits

Wild rice has a medium-glycemic index value of 57, just 2 points above low. When served with plenty of low-glycemic and high-fiber vegetables, the total recipe value is low glycemic.

Purple Cherry Coleslaw

A cherry-flavored crunchy purple salad.

1 (10-oz.) pkg. red cabbage slaw (about 6 cups)	**¾ cup walnut or olive oil**
1 green onion, chopped	**½ tsp. salt**
½ cup dried tart red cherries	**¼ tsp. freshly ground black pepper**
¼ cup red-wine vinegar	**1 TB. red cherry or raspberry preserves**

1. In a large salad bowl, combine slaw, green onion, and dried cherries.

2. In a small bowl, combine vinegar, oil, salt, pepper, and preserves. Toss desired amount of dressing with slaw mixture. Serve with salad tongs or a slotted spoon to drain any excess dressing.

Tasty Tidbits _____

Adding 1 tablespoon of preserves to a sauce or salad dressing barely increases the glycemic value, but adds a concentrated burst of flavor to your meal.

Yields 8 side-dish servings

Prep time: 15 minutes

Serving size: 1 cup cole-slaw

Each serving (salad):

Glycemic index: low

Glycemic load: 5

Calories: 54

Protein: 2 grams

Carbohydrates: 9 grams

Fiber: 2 grams

Fat: 0 grams

Saturated fat: 0 grams

Each serving (salad dressing per TB.):

Glycemic index: very low

Glycemic load: 0

Calories: 89

Protein: 0 grams

Carbohydrates: 2 grams

Fiber: 0 grams

Fat: 9 grams

Saturated fat: <1 gram

Coleslaw and Radish Salad

Yields 12 cups salad
Prep time: 30 minutes
Cook time: none
Serving size: 1 cup salad
Each serving (salad):
Glycemic index: very low
Glycemic load: <1
Calories: 28
Protein: 2 grams
Carbohydrates: 5 grams
Fiber: 3 grams
Fat: 0 grams
Saturated fat: 0 grams
Each serving (salad dressing per TB.):
Glycemic index: very low
Glycemic load: 0
Calories: 85
Protein: 0 grams
Carbohydrates: 1 gram
Fiber: 0 grams
Fat: 9 grams
Saturated fat: <1 gram

This coleslaw invites you to enjoy the tastes of jicama combined with the bright flavor of radishes.

¾ cup mayonnaise

¼ cup white-wine vinegar

1 TB. honey

2 tsp. celery seeds

½ tsp. salt

¼ tsp. freshly ground black pepper

1 lb. green cabbage, chopped, about 9 cups

2 medium carrots, finely shredded

1 cup shredded jicama

¼ cup shredded red radishes

1 cup snipped cilantro

1. For dressing: in a medium bowl, combine mayonnaise, vinegar, honey, celery seeds, salt, and pepper. Set aside.

2. In a large salad bowl, combine cabbage, carrots, jicama, radishes, and cilantro. Add desired amount of dressing and toss. Cover and refrigerate until serving time or up to 24 hours. Serve with a slotted spoon to let excess dressing drain from salad.

Glycemic Notes

Jicama is a crisp white tuber from Mexico with a neutral fresh taste. Peel before shredding.

Summer Vegetable Salad with Pasta

The fragrant taste of garlic and mustard adds heat to the fresh taste of zucchini, snap peas, and tomatoes.

¼ tsp. salt

8 oz. dried whole-grain penne pasta

1 TB. olive oil

6 to 8 cloves garlic, thinly sliced

1 medium zucchini, trimmed, cut into matchstick-size strips

8 oz. sugar snap peas

2 cups cherry tomatoes, halved

1 green onion, finely chopped

1 TB. white wine vinegar

1 TB. Dijon-style mustard

½ tsp. salt

¼ tsp. freshly ground black pepper

4 TB. olive oil

3 TB. chopped fresh parsley

Yields 8 cups salad
Prep time: 30 minutes
Cook time: 15 minutes
Serving size: 1 cup salad
Each serving (salad):
Glycemic index: low
Glycemic load: 9
Calories: 134
Protein: 4 grams
Carbohydrates: 26 grams
Fiber: 4 grams
Fat: 1.5 grams
Saturated fat: 0 grams
Each serving (salad dressing per TB.):
Glycemic index: very low
Glycemic load: 0
Calories: 72
Protein: 0 grams
Carbohydrates: <1 gram
Fat: 8 grams
Saturated fat: <1 gram

1. In a large saucepan over high heat, bring a large pot of water with ¼ teaspoon salt to boil. Add pasta. Undercook slightly to just before the al dente stage. Drain and rinse pasta under cold water; then drain again. Transfer pasta to a large salad bowl with a slotted spoon.

2. Heat 1 tablespoon olive oil in a large skillet over medium-high heat. Add garlic and cook 30 seconds. Add zucchini. Cook while stirring for 1 minute. Add snap peas. Cook 30 seconds. Stir in tomatoes. Cook 30 seconds. Add vegetable mixture to pasta in the bowl.

3. For salad dressing, combine green onions, vinegar, mustard, salt, and pepper. Slowly whisk in olive oil. Stir in parsley. Pour desired amount of dressing over pasta mixture; toss well. Serve with a slotted spoon.

4. Serve when slightly warm or chill before serving.

def•i•ni•tion

Al dente means "to the tooth" in Italian. To keep pasta low glycemic, undercook it. Stop the cooking process by flushing with cold water when the pasta is just the slightest bit crunchy. Test by sampling as the pasta cooks.

Arugula, Corn, and Papaya Salad

Yields 10 cups salad
Prep time: 20 minutes
Cook time: none
Serving size: 1²/₃ cup salad
Each serving (salad):
Glycemic index: low
Glycemic load: 7
Calories: 76
Protein: 3 grams
Carbohydrates: 16 grams
Fiber: 2 grams
Fat: <1 gram
Saturated fat: 0 grams
Each serving (salad dressing per TB.):
Glycemic index: very low
Glycemic load:
Calories: 90
Protein: 0 grams
Carbohydrates: 0 grams
Fat: 10 grams
Saturated fat: <1 gram

A tossed salad brings together the sweet tastes of corn and papaya, finished with a lime juice and curry dressing.

2 cups frozen corn	1 TB. fresh lime juice
2 small papayas	½ tsp. curry powder
1 red bell pepper	½ tsp. salt
6 cups fresh arugula	⅛ tsp. freshly ground black pepper
4 TB. olive oil	

1. Steam corn according to package directions. Cut papayas in half, remove seeds, and cut fruit into ¹/₄-inch slices. Cut red bell pepper into ¹/₂-inch pieces. Place corn, papayas, red bell pepper, and arugula into a salad bowl.

2. For dressing, combine olive oil, lime juice, curry, salt, and black pepper in a small bowl.

3. Pour desired amount of dressing on salad and toss gently. Serve with a slotted spoon to let dressing drain.

Beet Salad with Oranges

A tangy citrus dressing accents the unique anise taste of the fennel.

**4 red or golden beets, about
½ lb. with stems removed**

2 tsp. olive oil

2 medium oranges

1 fennel bulb

2 TB. olive oil

2 tsp. red wine vinegar

½ tsp. salt

¼ tsp. freshly ground pepper

8–12 red-leaf lettuce leaves

¼ cup toasted pinion nuts

1. Preheat the oven to 350°F.

2. Place beets in single layer in a shallow baking dish. Drizzle with 2 teaspoons olive oil and turn to coat. Roast, turning occasionally, until tender when pierced with a fork, about 1¹/₄ hours. When cool enough to handle, remove skins. Cut each beet into quarters.

3. Peel oranges and cut crosswise, removing pits. Place in a salad bowl.

4. Cut stems and rough base from fennel. Cut in half lengthwise, then cut fennel into ¹/₄-inch slices. Add to the bowl. Add beets.

5. Make salad dressing: in a jar with tight-fitting lid, shake together 2 tablespoons olive oil, red wine vinegar, salt, and pepper.

6. Place 2 lettuce leaves on each individual plate. Top with beet mixture, dividing evenly. Sprinkle with pinion nuts, dividing evenly. Top with desired amount of dressing. Serve.

Yields about 6 cups salad
Prep time: 20 minutes
Cook time: 1 hour 15 minutes
Serving size: 1 cup salad
Each serving (salad):
Glycemic index: low
Glycemic load: 5
Calories: 105
Protein: 2 grams
Carbohydrates: 13 grams
Fiber: 4 grams
Fat: 5 grams
Saturated fat: <1 gram
Each serving (salad dressing per TB.):
Glycemic index: very low
Glycemic load: 0
Calories: 99
Protein: 0 grams
Carbohydrates: 0 grams
Fat: 11 grams
Saturated fat: <1 gram

Tasty Tidbits

Fennel is favored for its mild anise or licorice taste. When sliced, it looks like a white version of celery. Serve raw in salads and cooked with fish or seafood.

Broccoli and Cauliflower Salad

The best deli-type salad we've ever eaten. It's crunchy, a bit sweet, and the bacon, cashews, and Parmesan flavors make you want to eat your broccoli.

Yields 8–9 cups salad
Prep time: 20 minutes
Cook time: none
Serving size: ¹/₂ cup
Each serving (salad):
Glycemic index: low
Glycemic load: 2
Calories: 174
Protein: 14 grams
Carbohydrates: 7 grams
Fiber: 3 grams
Fat: 10 grams
Saturated fat: 3 grams
Each serving (salad dressing per TB.):
Glycemic index: low
Glycemic load: 0
Calories: 96
Protein: 0 grams
Carbohydrates: 1.5 grams
Fat: 10 grams
Saturated fat: <1 gram

4 cups coarsely chopped fresh broccoli

4 cups coarsely chopped fresh cauliflower

5 celery ribs, sliced

1 (10-oz.) pkg. frozen peas, not cooked

1 cup coarsely chopped cashews

½ lb. bacon, fried and crumbled

1 cup mayonnaise

2 TB. honey

2 TB. red wine vinegar

¼ tsp. salt

¼ cup shredded Parmesan cheese

1. In a large bowl, toss together broccoli, cauliflower, celery, peas, pecans, and crumbled bacon.

2. In a small bowl, mix mayonnaise, honey, vinegar, and salt. Add desired amount of dressing to bowl of vegetables and stir gently to blend.

3. Sprinkle with Parmesan cheese. Refrigerate before serving. Serve with a slotted spoon.

Cabbage with Apples and Walnuts

The combination of brisk apples and earthy walnuts is dressed with a tangy, lemon-flavored vinegar-and-oil mixture.

½ head white cabbage

2 celery ribs, thinly sliced

2 carrots, coarsely grated

2 tsp. caraway seeds

1 apple such as Jonagold, Pink Lady, Gala, or Fuji, cored and chopped

½ cup walnuts, chopped

3 TB. olive oil

2 TB. white wine vinegar

1 tsp. grated lemon rind

¼ tsp. salt

⅛ tsp. freshly ground fresh pepper

1. Cut out and discard cabbage core. Finely shred cabbage leaves. Place in a large salad bowl.

2. Add celery, carrot, caraway seeds, apple, and walnuts.

3. In a small bowl, whisk olive oil, vinegar, lemon rind, salt, and pepper. Toss desired amount of dressing with salad. Serve with salad tongs or a slotted spoon.

 Tasty Tidbits _____

Serve this type of salad immediately after tossing with dressing. Otherwise, the apple could brown and the vegetables wilt.

Yields 6 cups salad
Prep time: 20 minutes
Cook time: none
Serving size: 1 cup salad
Each serving (salad):
Glycemic index: low
Glycemic load: 2
Calories: 98
Protein: 4 grams
Carbohydrates: 7 grams
Fiber: 4 grams
Fat: 6 grams
Saturated fat: <1 gram
Each serving (salad dressing per TB.):
Glycemic index: very low
Glycemic load: 0
Calories: 63
Protein: 0 grams
Carbohydrates: 0 grams
Fiber: 0
Fat: 7 grams
Saturated fat: <1 gram

Pine Nut Salad

Pine nuts lend an earthy mountain taste to blueberries and greens.

Yields 8 cups salad
Prep time: 15 minutes
Cook time: 10 minutes
Serving size: 1 cup salad
Each serving (salad):
Glycemic index: low
Glycemic load: 2
Calories: 141
Protein: 3 grams
Carbohydrates: 8 grams
Fiber: 2 grams
Fat: 3.5 grams
Saturated fat: <1 gram
Each serving (salad dressing per TB.):
Glycemic index: very low
Glycemic load: 0
Calories: 72
Protein: 0
Carbohydrates: <1 gram
Fiber: 0 grams
Fat: 8 grams
Saturated fat: <1 gram

¼ cup pine nuts

1 large head romaine lettuce, torn into pieces

¼ cup shaved Parmesan cheese

¼ cup dried blueberries

1 tsp. minced garlic

¼ tsp. salt

1 tsp. Dijon mustard

2 TB. white wine vinegar

¼ cup olive oil

1. Toast pine nuts in a skillet on medium-high heat. Stir until golden brown. Set aside.

2. In a large salad bowl, place romaine, Parmesan, pine nuts, and dried blueberries.

3. For salad dressing: in a small bowl, mix garlic and salt. Whisk in mustard, vinegar, and oil. Add desired amount of dressing to salad and toss gently. Serve with salad tongs or a slotted spoon.

Home-Cooked Goodness

Pinion nuts, also known as pine nuts, come from the cone of a pine tree. They have a distinctive taste and aroma of the forest. They're a beloved ingredient in many cuisines.

Caesar Salad

Garlic and salty anchovy paste combine with tangy lemon juice for a rich taste that dresses crisp and crunchy Romaine lettuce.

4 stone-ground bread, thickly sliced, without crusts

3 TB. olive oil

1 garlic clove, crushed

1 lb. Romaine lettuce (about 6 cups of leaves)

1 garlic clove, chopped

2 TB. lemon juice

dash of Worcestershire sauce

2 inches anchovy paste

⅓ cup olive oil

Salt

Freshly ground black pepper

¼ cup shaved Parmesan cheese

Yields 6 cups salad
Prep time: 15 minutes
Cook time: 5 minutes
Serving size: 1½ cups salad
Each serving (salad):
Glycemic index: low
Glycemic load: 6
Calories: 143
Protein: 5 grams
Carbohydrates: 14 grams
Fiber: 3 grams
Fat: 7.5 grams
Saturated fat: 1 gram
Each serving (salad dressing per TB.):
Glycemic index: very low
Glycemic load: 0
Calories: 81
Protein: 0 grams
Carbohydrates: 0 grams
Fiber: 0 grams
Fat: 9 grams
Saturated fat: 1 gram

1. Cut bread slices into 1-inch cubes. Heat 3 tablespoons olive oil and garlic clove in a large skillet over medium heat. Add bread cubes. Stir frequently until browned and fragrant. Remove from heat and let cool.

2. Wash lettuce leaves. Tear into bite-size pieces. Place in a large salad bowl.

3. To make dressing, in a separate small bowl, whisk garlic, lemon juice, Worcestershire sauce, anchovy paste, and ⅓ cup olive oil. Add salt and black pepper to taste.

4. Pour desired amount of dressing over salad greens. Toss well. Top with garlic croutons and shaved Parmesan cheese. Toss again.

5. Serve with salad tongs or a slotted spoon to drain excess dressing.

Variation: Serve without croutons to lower the glycemic index value to very low.

Home-Cooked Goodness

Parmesan cheese can be grated into very fine particles; shredded into thin slivers about ⅜-inch to ½-inch long; or shaved into thin slices that curl at the ends. Each adds an increasing intensity of flavor.

Classic Greek Salad

Savor the authentic fragrant and aromatic taste of the Greek islands: the olives, oregano, garlic, tomatoes, and feta cheese.

1 head Romaine lettuce	4 TB. feta cheese, crumbled
1 cucumber, halved lengthwise	½ tsp. dried oregano
	½ tsp. minced garlic
4 tomatoes	6 TB. white wine vinegar
1 green bell pepper, chopped in ½-inch pieces	⅓ cup olive oil
2 green onions, sliced	¼ tsp. salt
⅓ cup Kalamata olives	¼ tsp. freshly ground black pepper

1. Tear lettuce leaves into pieces. Place in a large salad bowl. Slice cucumber halves. Cut tomatoes into wedges.

2. Add cucumbers, tomatoes, peppers, sliced scallions, black olives, and feta cheese to the bowl.

3. To make dressing, put oregano, garlic, vinegar, olive oil, salt, and pepper into a small bowl and whisk well. Pour desired amount of dressing over salad and toss. Serve with a slotted spoon or salad tongs.

Tasty Tidbits

The Kalamata Greek black olives in this salad deliver a strong, deep, rich taste of a Greek salad. An ordinary black olive is milder and not as distinct.

Yields 8 cups salad

Prep time: 20 minutes
Cook time: none
Serving size: 2 cups salad
Each serving (salad):
Glycemic index: very low
Glycemic load: 0
Calories: 105
Protein: 7 grams
Carbohydrates: 8 grams
Fiber: 4 grams
Fat: 5.2 grams
Saturated fat: 2.5 grams

Each serving (salad dressing per TB.):
Glycemic index: very low
Glycemic load: 0
Calories: 49
Protein: 0 grams
Carbohydrates: 0 grams
Fiber: 0 grams
Fat: 5.5 grams
Saturated fat: <1 gram

Coleslaw with Carrots and Pineapple

Red and green cabbage blends with the fruity sweetness of pine-apple, raisins, and carrots.

2 cups coarsely shredded cabbage

1 cup coarsely shredded red cabbage

1 cup coarsely shredded carrots

1 (20-oz.) can pineapple chunks packed in water, well drained

⅓ cup toasted slivered almonds

¼ cup golden raisins

⅔ cup mayonnaise

⅔ cup yogurt (low fat plain)

1 tsp. grated onion

1 tsp. powdered ginger

2 TB. lemon juice

½ tsp. salt

Yields 8 cups coleslaw
Prep time: 20 minutes
Cook time: none
Serving size: 1 cup cole-slaw
Each serving (salad):
Glycemic index: low
Glycemic load: 7
Calories: 90
Protein: 3 grams
Carbohydrates: 15 grams
Fiber: 3 grams
Fat: 2 grams
Saturated fat: <1 gram
Each serving (salad dressing per TB.):
Glycemic index: very low
Glycemic load: 0
Calories: 62
Protein: 0 grams
Carbohydrates: 1 gram
Fiber: 0 grams
Fat: 6.5 grams
Saturated fat: 1 gram

1. Combine cabbage, carrots, pineapple, almonds, and raisins in a large salad bowl.

2. Make dressing by whisking together mayonnaise, yogurt, onion, ginger, lemon juice, and salt in a small bowl.

3. Toss cabbage mixture with desired amount of dressing. Chill 1 hour or longer.

4. Serve with a slotted spoon or salad tongs to drain excess dressing.

Cucumbers in Sour Cream

Yields 6 cups cucumbers in cream
Prep time: 15 minutes, plus 1 hour chill time
Cook time: none
Serving size: 1 cup cucumber in cream
Each serving (cucumbers):
Glycemic index: very low
Glycemic load: 0
Calories: 20
Protein: 1 gram
Carbohydrates: 4 grams
Fiber: 1.4 grams
Fat: 0 grams
Saturated fat: 0 grams
Each serving (salad dressing per TB.):
Glycemic index: very low
Glycemic load: 0
Calories: 14
Protein: 0 grams
Carbohydrates: <1 gram
Fiber: 0 grams
Fat: 1.5 grams
Saturated fat: <1 gram

The cucumbers soften as they blend with the salt and creamy, tangy sour cream.

6 cucumbers, medium-size

2 TB. red-wine vinegar

1 TB. chopped chives

½ tsp. salt

¼ tsp. freshly ground black pepper

⅓ cup yogurt

⅓ cup sour cream

1. Thinly slice cucumbers and place in a glass or ceramic bowl.

2. In a small bowl, mix red wine vinegar, chives, salt, and pepper. Pour on cucumbers.

3. Refrigerate 1 hour. When ready to serve, stir in desired amount of yogurt and sour cream.

Fennel Salad with Pomegranate and Orange

A colorful, festive salad with the subtle taste of fennel accented with the citrus of oranges and pomegranates.

2 large fennel bulbs, about 1½ lbs. total

2 oranges

4 TB. olive oil

2 TB. fresh lemon juice

⅛ tsp. freshly ground black pepper

8 lettuce leaves

4 TB. pomegranate seeds

1. Wash fennel bulbs and remove any brown or stringy outer leaves. Slice bulbs and stems into thin pieces. Place in a shallow serving bowl.

2. Peel oranges with a sharp knife, cutting away the white pith. Slice thinly crosswise. Cut each slice into thirds. Arrange over fennel, adding any juice from oranges.

3. To make dressing: mix oil, lemon juice, and pepper together. Pour desired amount of dressing on salad and mix well.

4. Place two lettuce leaves on each salad plate. Divide salad evenly among plates using a slotted spoon or salad tongs. Sprinkle each with 1 tablespoon pomegranate seeds.

Home-Cooked Goodness

Some grocery stores sell pomegranate seeds in tubs, saving you the work of separating the seeds from the pulp. The tubs are convenient for preparing salads and fruit dishes and for snacks.

Yields 4 cups salad
Prep time: 15 minutes
Cook time: none
Serving size: 1 cup salad
Each serving (salad):
Glycemic index: very low
Glycemic load: 4
Calories: 108
Protein: 3 grams
Carbohydrates: 24 grams
Fiber: 6 grams
Fat: 0 grams
Saturated fat: 0 grams
Each serving (salad dressing per TB.):
Glycemic index: very low
Glycemic load: none
Calories: 72
Protein: 0 grams
Carbohydrates: 0 grams
Fat: 8 grams
Fiber: 0 grams
Saturated fat: 1 gram

Jicama Pecan Salad

Yields 6 cups salad
Prep time: 20 minutes
Cook time: none
Serving size: 1 cup salad
Each serving (salad):
Glycemic index: very low
Glycemic load: 1
Calories: 91
Protein: 2 grams
Carbohydrates: 5 grams
Fiber: 3 grams
Fat: 7 grams
Saturated fat: <1 gram
Each serving (salad dressing per TB.):
Glycemic index: very low
Glycemic load: 0 grams
Calories: 72
Protein: 0 grams
Carbohydrates: 0 grams
Fiber: 0 grams
Fat: 8 grams
Saturated fat: 1 gram

A hot, spicy, crunchy jicama and bell pepper salad enhanced with a cilantro chile dressing.

2 cups jicama, peeled, cut into thin matchstick strips

3 small red, yellow, and/or green bell peppers, cut into thin matchstick strips

1 small red onion, thinly sliced and halved

¼ cup olive oil

⅓ cup chopped fresh cilantro

2 TB. red wine vinegar

1 small fresh jalapeño chile pepper, seeded and finely chopped

1 tsp. minced garlic

¼ tsp. freshly ground black pepper

⅛ tsp. salt

⅛ tsp. cayenne

¼ cup coarsely chopped pecans

1. In a large salad bowl, combine jicama strips, bell pepper, and onion slices.

2. In a screw-top jar, combine olive oil, cilantro, vinegar, chile pepper, garlic, black pepper, salt, and cayenne. Shake.

3. Pour desired amount dressing over jicama mixture. Toss.

4. Serve with a slotted spoon or salad tongs. Sprinkle with pecans before serving.

Variation: Substitute mild chiles for the jalapeño if you prefer less heat.

Chapter **18**

Vegetable Side Dishes

In This Chapter

- ◆ So many vegetables, so little time
- ◆ Seasonings make the vegetable
- ◆ Delicious in many ways

Vegetables are underrated. As the recipes in this chapter show, they are infinitely varied and simple to turn into interesting dishes. It's easy to eat 5–10 servings of vegetables and fruit every day.

Our vegetable recipes sport seasonings, spices, fruit, and nuts, such as cinnamon, basil, garlic, mint, horseradish, cherries, hazelnuts, and more. Dig in—you'll receive more than great taste and flavor. You'll also take in antioxidants, fiber, and other health-promoting nutrients as well.

Our recipes call for mostly fresh and frozen vegetables. These contain the most nutritional value. Occasionally, a recipe will call for canned vegetables for convenience, or because they aren't readily available in fresh or frozen form.

Sauté of Mushrooms

Buttery mushrooms flavored with garlic and fresh parsley.

Yields 2 cups mushrooms
Prep time: 10 minutes
Cook time: 20 minutes
Serving size: $^{1}/_{2}$ cup mushrooms
Each serving:
Glycemic index: very low
Glycemic load: 0
Calories: 102
Protein: 4 grams
Carbohydrates: 4 grams
Fiber: 1 gram
Fat: 6 grams
Saturated fat: 3.65 grams

2 TB. butter

1 lb. mushrooms, sliced

$^{1}/_{4}$ tsp. salt

$^{1}/_{8}$ tsp. ground black pepper

1 onion, finely chopped

1 tsp. minced garlic

1 TB. parsley, finely chopped

1. In a skillet over medium heat, melt 2 tablespoons butter, add mushrooms, and cook until golden brown. Add salt and pepper. Remove mushrooms from the skillet to a side dish.

2. Add 1 tablespoon butter to the skillet. Add onion, garlic, and parsley. Cook, stirring, until onion is translucent but not browned. Return mushrooms to the skillet and reheat. Serve, sprinkled with chopped parsley.

Broiled Tomatoes with Olives

Tomatoes with ham and green olives are flavored with basil.

Yields 12 tomato halves
Prep time: 15 minutes
Cook time: 10 minutes
Serving size: 2 tomato halves
Each serving:
Glycemic index: low
Glycemic load: 1
Calories: 162
Protein: 4 grams
Carbohydrates: 5 grams
Fiber: 2 grams
Fat: 14 grams
Saturated fat: 1 gram

6 medium tomatoes

$^{1}/_{2}$ cup lean 5 percent cooked ham, chopped

$^{1}/_{2}$ cup green olives, chopped

6 TB. fresh basil, chopped

6 TB. olive oil

1. Preheat the oven broiler to high.

2. Halve tomatoes and leave inverted a few minutes to drain. Arrange, cut-side up, in a shallow baking dish.

3. In a small bowl, mix ham and olives and place 1 rounded tablespoon mixture on each tomato half. Sprinkle with $^{1}/_{2}$ tablespoon basil and spoon $^{1}/_{2}$ tablespoon olive oil on top.

4. Broil about 3 inches from high broiler heat until tops are brown—about 10 minutes.

Butternut Squash with Tomato Bake

Rosemary adds full herbal flavor to the squash and herbed tomatoes.

Yields 6 cups squash with tomato bake
Prep time: 10 minutes
Cook time: 50 minutes
Serving size: 1 cup squash with tomato bake
Each serving:
Glycemic index: low
Glycemic load: 6
Calories: 149
Protein: 2 grams
Carbohydrates: 20 grams
Fiber: 3 grams
Fat: 7 grams
Saturated fat: <1 gram

1 butternut squash, peeled and seeded

3 TB. olive oil

2 (14-oz.) cans chopped tomatoes with herbs

2 tsp. dried rosemary

½ tsp. salt

¼ tsp. freshly ground black pepper

1. Preheat the oven to 325°F.

2. Slice squash into ³/₈-inch slices. In a large skillet over medium-high heat, sauté squash slices in olive oil until golden brown. Remove from the skillet to a side dish.

3. Add tomatoes and rosemary to the skillet and cook until heated. Add salt and pepper.

4. In a baking dish, repeatedly layer squash slices with tomato mixture, ending with tomato mixture.

5. Bake for 35 minutes.

Variation: Substitute acorn squash or pumpkin for butternut squash.

Home-Cooked Goodness

Use a vegetable peeler or small paring knife to peel butternut squash. It can be slippery, so wrap it with a kitchen towel to hold it securely.

Spaghetti Squash with Parmesan

Yields 1 spaghetti squash with ½ cup sauce
Prep time: 15 minutes **Cook time:** 40 minutes **Serving size:** ¼ squash with sauce
Each serving: Glycemic index: very low Glycemic load: 1 Calories: 209 Protein: 7 grams Carbohydrates: 10 grams Fiber: 2 grams Fat: 15.6 grams Saturated fat: 9.9 grams

Squash strands flavored with an oregano butter sauce and topped with fresh Parmesan.

1 spaghetti squash

¼ cup butter

1 tsp. dried parsley

1 tsp. dried oregano

1 tsp. minced garlic

1 tsp. lemon juice

¼ tsp. salt

⅛ tsp. freshly ground black pepper

¾ cup Parmesan cheese, freshly shredded

1. Preheat the oven to 350°F.

2. Cut squash in half lengthwise. Place halves, cut-side down, in a baking pan. Pour a little water around them and bake for 40 minutes, until tender.

3. In a small microwave bowl, melt butter. Stir in parsley, oregano, garlic, and lemon juice. Add salt and pepper.

4. Remove seeds from squash. With a fork, pull out the spaghetti-like strands and place in a serving bowl. Add butter mixture and toss. Sprinkle with Parmesan and serve.

Tasty Tidbits

Spaghetti squash is an excellent alternative to wheat spaghetti. It's lower glycemic, tastes slightly sweet, and is nutrient-dense while supplying antioxidants and vitamins.

Acorn Squash with Cherries

Acorn squash is baked with butter, walnuts, and cherries for a sweet, nutty flavor.

½ **cup orange juice**

¼ **cup tart red cherries, dried**

2 **acorn squash, halved and seeded**

2 **TB. butter**

¼ **cup walnuts, chopped**

½ **tsp. salt**

⅛ **tsp. freshly ground black pepper**

Yields 4 halves squash
Prep time: 15 minutes, plus 10 minutes stand time
Cook time: 1 hour
Serving size: ½ squash
Each serving:
Glycemic index: low
Glycemic load: 12
Calories: 270
Protein: 4 grams
Carbohydrates: 40 grams
Fiber: 10 grams
Fat: 10.5 grams
Saturated fat: 4.1 grams

1. Preheat the oven to 350°F. In a small saucepan over high heat, bring orange juice to a boil. Remove from heat. Add cherries and let stand 10 minutes.

2. Place acorn squash halves, cut-side up, in a baking dish. Place ½ tablespoon butter, 2 tablespoon walnuts, and ¼ orange juice with cherries mixture in each center. Sprinkle with salt and pepper. Bake for 1 hour.

Onions Baked in Their Skins

These onions are soft, sweet, and surprisingly delicious.

6 **medium onions**

6 **tsp. butter**

Salt and pepper

Yields 6 onions
Prep time: 5 minutes
Cook time: 1½ hours
Serving size: 1 onion
Each serving:
Glycemic index: very low
Glycemic load: 0
Calories: 78
Protein: 1 gram
Carbohydrates: 10 grams
Fiber: 2 grams
Fat: 3.8 grams
Saturated fat: 2.43 grams

1. Preheat the oven to 375°F.

2. Wash and dry onions. Bake until tender—about 1½ hours.

3. Cut a slice from root end of each onion and squeeze out center. Discard skins. Season with butter, salt, and pepper to taste.

Zucchini Pancakes

Zucchini is flavored with garlic, parsley, and Parmesan.

Yields 12 pancakes
Prep time: 10 minutes
Cook time: 12 minutes
Serving size: 2 pancakes
Each serving:
Glycemic index: low
Glycemic load: 2
Calories: 92
Protein: 8 grams
Carbohydrates: 7 grams
Fiber: 2 grams
Fat: 8 grams
Saturated fat: 1.5 grams

6 medium unpeeled zucchini, grated

3 eggs, lightly beaten

4 TB. Hi-Maize Resistant Starch

½ tsp. fresh parsley, minced

5 TB. Parmesan cheese, shredded

½ tsp. salt

¼ tsp. pepper

1 tsp. minced garlic

2 TB. olive oil

1. In a large mixing bowl, combine zucchini with eggs, Hi-Maize, parsley, Parmesan, salt, pepper, and garlic. Stir to blend. With your hands, form mixture into 12 patties, 3 inches in diameter.

2. In a large skillet, heat olive oil over medium-high heat. Cook pancakes 3 minutes per side. Drain on paper towels.

Peas with Pimentos

A crunchy dish flavored with zesty sun-dried tomatoes and lemon.

Yields 4 cups peas
Prep time: 10 minutes
Cook time: none
Serving size: ⅔ cup peas
Each serving:
Glycemic index: low
Glycemic load: 6
Calories: 116
Protein: 6 grams
Carbohydrates: 15 grams
Fiber: 4 grams
Fat: 8 grams
Saturated fat: 5 grams

1 cup sour cream

1 tsp. salt

¼ tsp. freshly ground black pepper

¼ tsp. dried lemon peel

¼ tsp. garlic powder

2 (10-oz.) pkgs. frozen peas, thawed

1 (2-oz.) jar chopped pimento

1 TB. chopped sun-dried tomatoes, packed in oil

¼ cup red onion, minced

1. In a medium mixing bowl, combine sour cream, salt, pepper, lemon peel, garlic powder, peas, pimentos, sun-dried tomatoes, and red onion.

2. Mix thoroughly and refrigerate overnight.

Broccoli with Blue Cheese Sauce

Broccoli topped with blue cheese.

1¼ lbs. fresh broccoli	3 oz. low-fat cream cheese
2 TB. olive oil	⅓ cup blue cheese, crumbled
2 TB. flour	¼ cup walnuts, chopped
1 cup skim milk	

1. Steam broccoli over boiling water in a saucepan fitted with a steamer. Cook until just tender. Remove from heat and keep warm.

2. In a medium saucepan, heat olive oil over medium heat. Stir in flour and heat until bubbly. Lower heat and slowly add milk, stirring until mixture thickens. Add cream cheese and blue cheese. Stir until cheese melts.

3. Place broccoli on serving platter. Pour sauce over broccoli. Top with walnuts and serve.

Yields 1¼ lbs. broccoli with 2 cups cheese sauce
Prep time: 5 minutes
Cook time: 5 minutes
Serving size: 1 cup broccoli and ¼ cup sauce
Each serving:
Glycemic index: very low
Glycemic load: <1
Calories: 133
Protein: 5 grams
Carbohydrates: 8 grams
Fiber: 3 grams
Fat: 9 grams
Saturated fat: 2.9 grams

Horseradish Carrots

Sweet carrots are given extra punch with tangy horseradish.

4 cups carrot sticks	1 tsp. salt
¼ cup reserved water	¼ tsp. freshly ground black pepper
2 TB. horseradish	
½ cup mayonnaise	

1. Preheat the oven to 375°F.

2. In a large saucepan over medium-high heat, add water to carrots and cook until just tender. Drain. Reserve ¼ cup cooking water.

3. Place carrots in a shallow 9×9-inch glass baking dish. In a small mixing bowl, mix reserved cooking water, horseradish, mayonnaise, salt, and pepper.

4. Pour mixture over carrots. Bake for 20 minutes until top is lightly browned.

Yields 4 cups carrots
Prep time: 10 minutes
Cook time: 25 minutes
Serving size: ⅔ cup carrots
Each serving:
Glycemic index: low
Glycemic load: 2
Calories: 154
Protein: 2 grams
Carbohydrates: 5 grams
Fiber: 2 grams
Fat: 14 grams
Saturated fat: 2 grams

Brussels Sprouts with Tomatoes

Yields 6 cups Brussels sprouts with onions and tomatoes

Prep time: 10 minutes

Cook time: 20 minutes

Serving size: 1 cup Brussels sprouts, tomatoes, and onions

Each serving:

Glycemic index: very low

Glycemic load: <1

Calories: 113

Protein: 5 grams

Carbohydrates: 8 grams

Fiber: 3 grams

Fat: 6.8 grams

Saturated fat: 3.5 grams

Bacon and onions flavor the Brussels sprouts, which are topped with sour cream, creating a rich taste.

1 lb. Brussels sprouts, trimmed and halved	**2 small tomatoes, seeded and diced**
4 strips bacon	**¼ tsp. salt**
1 TB. butter	**⅛ tsp. freshly ground black pepper**
1 medium yellow onion, chopped	**6 TB. sour cream**

1. In a large saucepan fitted with a vegetable steamer, over high heat, steam sprouts until tender—about 6–10 minutes—and set aside.

2. In a medium skillet over medium-high heat, cook bacon until crisp. Drain and set aside. Discard all but 2 teaspoons drippings.

3. Add butter and onion to the skillet. Reduce heat to medium and cook until onion is transparent. Crumble bacon and add to onion. Stir in tomatoes. Add salt and pepper. Warm Brussels sprouts in mixture and serve with dollop of sour cream.

Variation: For lower fat, use half the bacon, butter, and sour cream. Results: 83 calories, 3.4 grams fat, 1.75 grams saturated fat.

Home-Cooked Goodness

Turkey bacon provides a delicious alternative to regular bacon. It has fewer calories, usually less fat—check the label—and provides a substantial meaty taste.

Mock Garlic Mashed Potatoes

Cauliflower enhanced with the flavors of sour cream and garlic.

3 cups cauliflower, chopped

1 TB. butter

½ tsp. minced garlic

¼ cup sour cream

¼ tsp. salt

⅛ tsp. freshly ground black pepper

1. In a saucepan fitted with a vegetable steamer, over high heat, steam cauliflower until soft enough to mash.

2. Place cauliflower in a food processor fitted with a chopping blade. Add butter, garlic, and sour cream, and blend until texture of mashed potatoes.

3. Stir in salt and pepper. Serve.

Variation: Increase garlic if you like a stronger taste. Omit garlic if you prefer. Top with Parmesan cheese for a richer taste.

Yields 3 cups potatoes
Prep time: 10 minutes
Cook time: 5 minutes
Serving size: ½ cup potatoes
Each serving:
Glycemic index: very low
Glycemic load: 0
Calories: 52
Protein: 1 gram
Carbohydrates: 3 grams
Fiber: 1 gram
Fat: 3.68 grams
Saturated fat: 2.26 grams

Tasty Tidbits _____

Believe it or not, mock mashed potatoes taste like mashed white potatoes, but offer several important nutritional advantages: they don't contain starch, they're low glycemic, they offer antioxidants and vitamins, and they count as one of your 5–10 daily servings of vegetables.

Peas with Mint and Ricotta

Yields 2¼ cups peas
Prep time: 15 minutes
Cook time: 10 minutes
Serving size: ¹/₂ cup peas
Each serving:
Glycemic index: low
Glycemic load: 4
Calories: 139
Protein: 8 grams
Carbohydrates: 11 grams
Fiber: 3 grams
Fat: 7 grams
Saturated fat: 2.3 grams

Mint lends an aromatic, sweet taste to the peas, accented with salty bacon and creamy Italian ricotta cheese.

1 (10-oz.) pkg. frozen peas

2 thin slices bacon, chopped

1 TB. olive oil

1 tsp. raspberry vinegar

¹/₂ tsp. salt

¹/₂ tsp. freshly ground black pepper

2 TB. fresh mint, finely chopped

¼ cup ricotta cheese, crumbled

1. In a saucepan fitted with a vegetable steamer, over high heat, steam peas until barely tender—about 6–10 minutes. Drain. Run cold water over peas to cool. Drain. Set aside.

2. In a skillet over medium heat, cook bacon, stirring until lightly crisp—about 4–5 minutes. With a slotted spoon, transfer to paper towels to drain.

3. In a large mixing bowl, whisk together olive oil, vinegar, salt, and pepper. Add peas, bacon, and mint, turning to coat. Stir in ricotta.

4. Transfer salad to a serving bowl.

Tasty Tidbits

Peas are often ignored when choosing vegetables for dinner, but they always provide color and a creamy taste to your meal.

Lemon Carrots

A light sauce flavored with herbs and lemon lends a tangy taste to sweet carrots.

2¼ cups water

1 lb. carrots, thinly sliced

½ tsp. dried parsley

½ tsp. dried thyme

1 bay leaf

1 TB. freshly squeezed lemon juice

½ tsp. dried lemon peel

¼ tsp. salt

⅛ tsp. freshly ground black pepper

1½ TB. butter

1 TB. all-purpose flour

Yields 3 cups carrots
Prep time: 10 minutes
Cook time: 15 minutes
Serving size: ³/₄ cup carrots

Each serving:
Glycemic index: low
Glycemic load: 6
Calories: 91
Protein: 1 gram
Carbohydrates: 12 grams
Fiber: 3 grams
Fat: 4.3 grams
Saturated fat: 2.75 grams

1. In a large saucepan over high heat, bring water to a boil, then add carrots, parsley, thyme, bay leaf, lemon juice and peel, salt, and pepper. Simmer until carrots are tender. Remove carrots using a slotted spoon. Keep warm.

2. Boil the cooking liquid hard until it has reduced to about 1¹/₄ cups. Discard bay leaf.

3. Mash 1 tablespoon butter and flour together in a bowl. Gradually whisk into simmering, reduced cooking liquid, whisking well after each addition. Simmer for about 3 minutes, until sauce has thickened.

4. Return carrots to the saucepan to heat thoroughly. Remove from heat. Stir in remaining butter and serve immediately.

Beets in Citrus Sauce

Beets fragrant with allspice and flavored with a citrus tang.

Yields 4 cups beets	

Prep time: 20 minutes

Cook time: 20 minutes

Serving size: 1/2 cup beets

Each serving:

Glycemic index: medium

Glycemic load: 9

Calories: 95

Protein: 2 grams

Carbohydrates: 15 grams

Fiber: 3 grams

Fat: 2.87 grams

Saturated fat: 1.8 grams

2 lbs. beets

1 TB. vinegar

3/4 cup fresh orange juice

3 TB. lemon juice

2 tsp. orange rind, grated

1/8 tsp. ground allspice

1/2 TB. honey

2 TB. butter

1. Scrub beets and cut off tops, leaving 1-inch greens attached. Place in a saucepan. Add boiling water until covered. Add vinegar and cook until tender—about 20 minutes.

2. Drain beets, reserving some liquid. Skin beets, then slice and keep them warm.

3. Strain enough reserved beet liquid to yield 1/4 cup. Combine with orange juice, lemon juice, orange rind, and allspice.

4. Bring to a boil, stirring. Add honey and butter and mix. Pour over beets.

Home-Cooked Goodness

Use 2 (16-oz.) cans of sliced beets if you're pressed for time and you'll shorten the total preparation time by 20 minutes.

Sweet and Sour Cabbage

Boiled cabbage is made sweet and tangy with honey and vinegar.

½ cup cider vinegar

2 TB. honey

1 quart water

1 large head cabbage,
coarsely shredded

2 TB. flour

½ tsp. caraway seeds

2 TB. butter

Yields 3 cups cabbage
Prep time: 10 minutes
Cook time: 25–30 minutes
Serving size: ¹/₂ cup cabbage
Each serving:
Glycemic index: low
Glycemic load: 4
Calories: 132
Protein: 3 grams
Carbohydrates: 21 grams
Fiber: 4 grams
Fat: 4 grams
Saturated fat: 2.4 grams

1. In a large saucepan, combine vinegar, honey, and water. Add cabbage. Over high heat, bring to a boil and boil vigorously, uncovered, for 25 minutes.

2. Mix flour with a little cold water and stir into hot cabbage. Add caraway seeds. Cook, stirring until mixture thickens. Remove to a serving bowl. Top with butter.

Variation: Heat up the cabbage by substituting ¹/₂ teaspoon chili powder for the caraway seeds.

Summer Vegetables Braise

Carrots, peas, and baby corn are gently flavored with parsley and lime juice.

8 oz. baby carrots

1½ cups sugar snap peas or snow peas

4 oz. baby corn cobs

6 TB. water

2 tsp. lime juice

½ tsp. salt

⅛ tsp. freshly ground black pepper

1 TB. chopped fresh parsley

Yields 4 cups vegetables
Prep time: 10 minutes
Cook time: 10 minutes
Serving size: 1 cup vegetables
Each serving:
Glycemic index: low
Glycemic load: 2
Calories: 36
Protein: 1 gram
Carbohydrates: 8 grams
Fiber: 3 grams
Fat: 0 grams
Saturated fat: 0 grams

1. In a large saucepan over medium-high heat, add carrots, peas, baby corn cobs, water, and lime juice. Bring to a boil.

2. Cover the saucepan and reduce heat. Simmer for 6–8 minutes, shaking pan occasionally, until vegetables are just tender.

3. Season vegetables with salt, pepper, and parsley.

Rosemary Roasted Vegetables

Green beans and Brussels sprouts are deliciously roasted and flavored with rosemary sprigs.

Yields 8 cups vegetables
Prep time: 15 minutes
Cook time: 20 minutes
Serving size: ³/₄ cup vegetables
Each serving:
Glycemic index: very low
Glycemic load: 0
Calories: 54
Protein: 2 grams
Carbohydrates: 7 grams
Fiber: 3 grams
Fat: 1.9 grams
Saturated fat: 1.2 grams

4 cups (1 lb.) fresh Brussels sprouts

4 cups (12 oz.) fresh, whole green beans

1 bunch green onions (6), trimmed and sliced

12 fresh rosemary sprigs

2 TB. olive oil

Salt and freshly ground black pepper

Juice from 1 lemon

1. Preheat the oven to 425°F.

2. Cut large Brussels sprouts in half. In a large covered saucepan fitted with a vegetable steamer, over high heat, steam Brussels sprouts for 3 minutes. Add beans. Steam for 5 minutes. Remove from heat.

3. Place Brussels sprouts and beans in a shallow roasting pan. Add green onions and rosemary sprigs. Toss to combine.

4. Drizzle vegetable mixture with olive oil. Sprinkle with salt and pepper. Roast, uncovered, about 20 minutes or until vegetables are crisp-tender. Transfer to a platter. Squeeze lemon juice over vegetables.

Tasty Tidbits

Roasting keeps vegetables crisp and crunchy and lets them retain their individual flavors.

Green Beans with Herb Sauce

Tomatoes, basil, and garlic flavor the herb sauce poured over the beans.

2 lbs. green beans	3 TB. celery, chopped
3 TB. olive oil	2 TB. parsley, chopped
1 TB. butter	1 tsp. red wine vinegar
1 onion, chopped	¼ tsp. dried basil
1 tsp. minced garlic	½ tsp. salt
2 tomatoes, peeled, seeded, and chopped	⅛ tsp. freshly ground black pepper

Yields 8 cups beans
Prep time: 15 minutes
Cook time: 10 minutes
Serving size: 1 cup beans
Each serving:
Glycemic index: very low
Glycemic load: 0
Calories: 98
Protein: 2 grams
Carbohydrates: 8 grams
Fiber: 4 grams
Fat: 6.5 grams
Saturated fat: 1.6 grams

1. In a large saucepan fitted with a vegetable steamer, over high heat, steam green beans until slightly tender—about 5 minutes. Remove from heat and keep warm.

2. Heat oil and butter in a small skillet over medium heat. Sauté onion and garlic until tender. Add tomatoes, celery, parsley, vinegar, basil, salt, and pepper. Bring to a boil and simmer 10 minutes.

3. Pour tomato mixture over hot beans.

Glycemic Notes

When steaming vegetables, be sure to add enough water to the saucepan. Otherwise, your saucepan could overheat and burn.

Green Beans with Hazelnuts

Lemon flavors this unique combination of green beans and toasted hazelnuts.

2 lbs. green beans, trimmed	1 tsp. lemon peel, grated
½ cup chopped hazelnuts (filberts)	½ tsp. salt
2 TB. butter	¼ tsp. freshly ground black pepper

1. Bring a saucepan fitted with a vegetable steamer to a boil over high heat. Add beans and steam for 3 minutes.

2. In a large skillet over medium-high heat, sauté hazelnuts in butter for 3 minutes to toast nuts. Add green beans, lemon peel, salt, and pepper. Cook, stirring, for 5 minutes.

Yields 8 cups green beans

Prep time: 10 minutes

Cook time: 8 minutes

Serving size: 1 cup green beans

Each serving:

Glycemic index: very low

Glycemic load: 0

Calories: 109

Protein: 3 grams

Carbohydrates: 8 grams

Fiber: 4 grams

Fat: 7.25 grams

Saturated fat: 2.15 grams

Cinnamon Beans

The fragrant and zesty flavor of cinnamon spices up green beans.

1 TB. butter	¾ cup water
¼ cup chopped onion	⅛ tsp. salt
½ tsp. ground cinnamon	⅛ tsp. freshly ground black pepper
1 lb. fresh green beans	
1 lb. fresh wax beans	2 TB. tomato paste

1. In a skillet over medium-high heat, melt butter and sauté onion with cinnamon until onion is transparent.

2. Stir in beans, water, salt, and pepper. Heat to boiling, then reduce heat and simmer 20 minutes, or until beans are tender. Gently mix in tomato paste.

Yields 4 cups beans

Prep time: 10 minutes

Cook time: 25 minutes

Serving size: ½ cup beans

Each serving:

Glycemic index: very low

Glycemic load: 0

Calories: 53

Protein: 2 grams

Carbohydrates: 8 grams

Fiber: 4 grams

Fat: 1.5 grams

Saturated fat: 1 gram

Home-Cooked Goodness

Serve cinnamon beans with your favorite entrées—they blend well with many cuisines and tastes.

Asparagus with Tarragon Butter

Tarragon in lemon butter flavors the asparagus bunches.

1¼ lbs. fresh asparagus

4 TB. butter

2 TB. fresh tarragon, chopped

½ lemon rind, grated

1 TB. lemon juice

Salt and black pepper

Yields 4 bunches asparagus
Prep time: 10 minutes
Cook time: 6–8 minutes
Serving size: About ³/₄ cup asparagus
Each serving:
Glycemic index: very low
Glycemic load: 0
Calories: 140
Protein: 3 grams
Carbohydrates: 6 grams
Fiber: 3 grams
Fat: 11.5 grams
Saturated fat: 7.3 grams

1. Trim woody ends from asparagus spears. Place bundles of asparagus in a large skillet with 1 inch boiling water. Cover and cook for 6–8 minutes, until asparagus is tender but still firm. Drain well. Arrange asparagus spears equally on four serving plates.

2. In a small microwavable bowl, mix butter, tarragon, parsley, lemon rind, lemon juice, salt, and pepper. Microwave 30 seconds until butter melts. Stir sauce. Pour sauce over asparagus.

Baked Fennel with Parmesan Cheese

Anise-flavored fennel is accented with Parmesan and butter.

4 fennel bulbs, washed and cut in half

4 TB. butter

½ cup Parmesan cheese, freshly shredded

Yields 4 fennel bulbs
Prep time: 10 minutes
Cook time: 25 minutes
Serving size: ¹/₂ bulb each
Each serving:
Glycemic index: very low
Glycemic load: 0
Calories: 86
Protein: 2 grams
Carbohydrates: 5 grams
Fiber: 2 grams
Fat: 6.45 grams
Saturated fat: 4.08 grams

1. Preheat the oven to 400°F.

2. Fit a large saucepan with a vegetable steamer. Fill to bottom with water. Bring to boil. Place fennel bulbs in basket and steam until just tender.

3. Cut fennel bulbs lengthwise into 4–6 pieces. Place in a shallow, buttered baking dish.

4. Dot with butter. Sprinkle with Parmesan. Bake until cheese is golden brown—about 20 minutes. Serve at once.

Steamed Artichokes
with Lemon Butter

Succulent artichokes flavored with garlic and lemon.

4 globe artichokes	**½ cup butter**
1 garlic clove	**¼ cup fresh lemon juice**
1 tsp. salt	

Yields 4 artichokes
Prep time: 10 minutes
Cook time: 40–60 minutes
Serving size: 1 artichoke, plus 2 TB. butter
Each serving:
Glycemic index: very low
Glycemic load: 0
Calories: 275
Protein: 4 grams
Carbohydrates: 13 grams
Fiber: 7 grams
Fat: 23 grams
Saturated fat: 14.5 grams

1. Wash artichokes, then trim stems and remove loose leaves. Cut off 1 inch from each top. Snip off sharp leaf tips.

2. In a large saucepan with about 1 inch water, place garlic clove and salt. Place steamer basket in saucepan and add artichokes. Bring water to boiling. Cover, reduce heat, and simmer for 40–60 minutes. Artichokes are done when you can easily pull a leaf from center. Remove from the saucepan with tongs or a slotted spoon.

3. While artichokes are cooling, melt butter in a small microwavable bowl. Stir in lemon juice.

4. Serve with a side bowl for butter sauce, and another bowl to catch leaf remnants.

Home-Cooked Goodness

To eat artichokes, pull off one leaf at a time. Dip base of leaf into melted butter. Draw through your teeth, scraping off the tender flesh. Discard remainder of leaf. Continue removing leaves until the fuzzy choke appears. Scoop out with a spoon. Eat the heart with a fork, dipping each piece into sauce.

Glycemic Notes

If you're watching your saturated fat intake, eat the butter sauce sparingly. Dip each leaf in the sauce and tap to remove excess butter before eating. Plan to have sauce left over.

Chapter 19

Potatoes and Sweet Potatoes

In This Chapter

- ◆ Preparing low- and medium-glycemic potatoes
- ◆ Many variations of sweet potatoes
- ◆ Using red potatoes in your recipes

We all love potatoes, and in this chapter you'll find plenty of mouth-watering low- and medium-glycemic recipes for "America's favorite vegetable."

You'll find potato salads, baked fries, Holiday casseroles, twice-baked potatoes—all of your favorites and some new choices, too.

Potato Salad with Eggs

The flavor of the potatoes shines with a lightly seasoned dressing.

Yields 5 cups salad
Prep time: 15 minutes
Cook time: 20 minutes
Serving size: 1/2 cup salad
Each serving:
Glycemic index: medium
Glycemic load: 10
Calories: 250
Protein: 3 grams
Carbohydrates: 16 grams
Fiber: 2 grams
Fat: 9 grams
Saturated fat: 2 grams

2 lbs. red potatoes, scrubbed or peeled

1/4 tsp. salt

1 TB. onion, finely chopped

2 hard-boiled eggs, peeled and chopped

1 1/4 cups mayonnaise

1/2 tsp. minced garlic

2 TB. fresh lemon juice

1 tsp. fresh lemon peel, grated

4 TB. fresh parsley, chopped

1/2 tsp. salt

1/4 tsp. freshly ground black pepper

1. Bring potatoes with salt to a boil in a saucepan over high heat. Lower heat and simmer for 20 minutes. Drain and cool. Cut potatoes into large cubes and place in a mixing bowl. Add onion and eggs.

2. Mix mayonnaise, garlic, lemon juice, lemon peel, parsley, salt, and pepper in a small bowl. Pour over potatoes and stir gently to mix.

Home-Cooked Goodness

To peel or not to peel? Which do you choose? Scrubbed, unpeeled potatoes add more color and texture to potato salad. And they provide more nutritional fiber. Peeled potatoes provide consistent color and texture. Whichever you prefer makes little to no difference nutritionally.

Scalloped Carrots and Potatoes

Delicate, creamy carrots and potatoes flavored with nutmeg.

2 cups white potatoes, sliced thick

4 cups carrots, sliced thick

¼ cup Hi-Maize Resistant Starch

¼ cup butter

1 tsp. salt

¼ tsp. ground black pepper

¼ tsp. nutmeg

2 cups milk

Yields 9 servings
Prep time: 15 minutes
Cook time: 1 hour
Serving size: 1 (3×4-inch) square
Each serving:
Glycemic index: medium
Glycemic load: 9
Calories: 143
Protein: 4 grams
Carbohydrates: 16 grams
Fiber: 2 grams
Fat: 7 grams
Saturated fat: 4 grams

1. Preheat the oven to 400°F.

2. Make a layer of ¹/₂ the potatoes in the bottom of a greased 9×13-inch baking dish. Top with ¹/₂ the carrots.

3. Sprinkle with ¹/₂ the Hi-Maize and dot with ¹/₂ the butter. Season with ¹/₂ salt, pepper, and nutmeg.

4. Make a second layer of remaining carrots and another of remaining potatoes. Sprinkle with remaining Hi-Maize, dot with remaining butter, and season with remaining seasonings. Pour cream or milk over all and bake about 1 hour, until browned and tender.

Tasty Tidbits _____

You can use flour in place of the Hi-Maize Resistant Starch if you don't have the latter on hand. Using flour in this recipe will only slightly raise the glycemic index and load, because it's not a major ingredient like the white potatoes and carrots.

Home-Cooked Goodness _____

Carrots were once thought to be high glycemic. They don't deserve this bad reputation. Instead, they are low glycemic at 47.

Mashed Roasters

Yields 6 servings
Prep time: 15 minutes
Cook time: 30 minutes
Serving size: ³/₄ cup
Each serving:
Glycemic index: medium
Glycemic load: 15
Calories: 183
Protein: 4 grams
Carbohydrates: 26 grams
Fiber: 3 grams
Fat: 7 grams
Saturated fat: .57 grams

Coarsely mashed red potatoes are flavored with oregano.

2½ lbs. small red potatoes, halved

3 TB. olive oil

2 tsp. dried oregano, crushed

½ tsp. salt

¼ tsp. freshly ground black pepper

About 1 cup milk, warmed

1. Preheat the oven to 450°F. Lightly oil a 15×10×1-inch baking pan.

2. Arrange potatoes in a single layer in the pan. Cut any large potato pieces in half again. Sprinkle with olive oil, oregano, salt, and pepper. Toss to coat.

3. Roast potatoes, uncovered, for 30 minutes or until tender and browned, stirring twice during roasting.

4. Transfer potatoes and any pan drippings to a large bowl. Mash slightly with a fork or potato masher. Stir in enough milk to desired consistency.

Variation: Substitute tarragon, thyme, or parsley for the oregano.

 Tasty Tidbits

Mash these roasters to your preference—smooth or chunky. Serve with gravy, au jus, or butter.

Cheese Potato Bake

Swiss cheese flavors the potatoes, accented with a light onion taste.

6 medium-size white pota-toes, sliced	¼ tsp. ground black pepper
1½ cups Gruyère or Swiss cheese, shredded	2 TB. onion, finely grated
1 tsp. salt	1 cup heavy cream
	1 tsp. paprika

1. Preheat the oven to 325°F.

2. In a greased 9×13-inch baking pan, place ⅓ of potatoes. Sprinkle with ⅓ cheese, salt, pepper, and onion.

3. Repeat with 2 more layers of potatoes, cheese, and seasonings. Pour 1 cup heavy cream over all. Sprinkle with paprika and bake 2 hours.

Yields 6 cups bake
Prep time: 15 minutes
Cook time: 2 hours
Serving size: ½ cup bake
Each serving:
Glycemic index: medium
Glycemic load: 10
Calories: 120
Protein: 7 grams
Carbohydrates: 15 grams
Fiber: 1 gram
Fat: 10 grams
Saturated fat: 7 grams

Cheese Sweet Potato Sticks

Baked potato sticks seasoned with Parmesan and paprika.

4 large sweet potatoes	¼ cup butter, melted
¼ tsp. garlic powder	¼ cup Parmesan cheese, shredded
¼ tsp. paprika	

1. Preheat the oven to 450°F.

2. Wash potatoes. Don't peel. Cut into strips ⅜-inch wide.

3. Place potatoes in a resealable plastic bag. Add garlic powder and paprika. Toss to blend.

4. Arrange a single layer of potatoes in a shallow, greased baking pan. Brush with melted butter.

5. Bake 20–30 minutes, turning occasionally, until potatoes are crisp and browned. Sprinkle with Parmesan cheese.

Yields 8 cups sticks
Prep time: 15 minutes
Cook time: 20–30 min-utes
Serving size: 1 cup sticks
Each serving:
Glycemic index: low
Glycemic load: 13
Calories: 199
Protein: 4 grams
Carbohydrates: 30 grams
Fiber: 6 grams
Fat: 7 grams
Saturated fat: 4 grams

French Potato Salad

Tarragon and Dijon mustard give this red potato salad an herbal kick.

Yields 4 cups salad
Prep time: 15 minutes
Cook time: 10 minutes
Serving size: ¹/₂ cup salad
Each serving:
Glycemic index: medium
Glycemic load: 12
Calories: 146
Protein: 3 grams
Carbohydrates: 20 grams
Fiber: 2 grams
Fat: 6 grams
Saturated fat: <1 gram

8 medium-size red potatoes
Boiling salted water
1 tsp. salt
½ tsp. ground black pepper
¼ cup white wine vinegar
2 TB. beef broth

1 TB. Dijon mustard
¼ cup dry white wine
½ TB. tarragon, chopped
3 TB. parsley, chopped
¼ cup olive oil

1. In a large saucepan over high heat, cook potatoes in boiling salted water until tender but still firm. Cut potatoes into ¹/₄-inch-thick slices. Place in a salad bowl.

2. In a small bowl, combine salt, pepper, vinegar, broth, mustard, and wine. Stir until salt dissolves. Add tarragon, parsley, and olive oil and mix well. Pour over potatoes and toss gently.

Sweet Potato Peanut Casserole

Mashed sweet potatoes are flavored with peanuts and coconut.

Yields 9–10 cups casserole
Prep time: 35 minutes
Cook time: 25 minutes, plus 30–35 minutes bake time
Serving size: ³/₄ cup casserole
Each serving:
Glycemic index: low
Glycemic load: 11
Calories: 213
Protein: 8 grams
Carbohydrates: 25 grams
Fiber: 4 grams
Fat: 9 grams
Saturated fat: 6 grams

4 lbs. sweet potatoes, peeled and cut into quarters
2 TB. molasses
2 TB. honey
½ cup butter, cut up
¼ cup milk

4 eggs, lightly beaten
3–4 TB. lemon juice
½ cup peanut butter
2 TB. salted peanuts, coarsely chopped
3 TB. shredded coconut

1. In a large saucepan over medium-high heat, place potatoes in enough boiling salted water to cover. Boil for 25–30 minutes, covered, or until tender. Drain and return to the pan.

2. Preheat the oven to 350°F.

3. Slightly mash potatoes with a potato masher. Stir in molasses, honey, butter, milk, eggs, lemon juice, and peanut butter. Transfer sweet potato mixture to a greased 3-quart rectangular baking dish. Top with peanuts and coconut. Bake, uncovered, for 30–35 minutes, or until heated through.

Hot Apple and Potato Salad

Golden raisins and apples add sweetness balanced with savory bacon and tangy lemon.

½ cup golden raisins

1 cup boiling water

4 slices bacon

4 TB. vinegar

1 tsp. lemon rind, grated

2 TB. honey

3 cups cooked red potatoes, sliced

1 cup celery, diced

2 TB. parsley, chopped

2 tsp. salt

¼ tsp. ground black pepper

3 unpeeled apples, cored and sliced (3 cups)

Yields 7 cups salad
Prep time: 20 minutes
Cook time: 20 minutes
Serving size: Scant ⅔ cup salad
Each serving:
Glycemic index: low
Glycemic load: 12
Calories: 109
Protein: 3 g
Carbohydrates: 22 grams
Fiber: 2 grams
Fat: 1 gram
Saturated fat: <1 gram

1. Place raisins in a bowl. Pour boiling water over raisins. Let stand 3 minutes. Drain.

2. In a large skillet over medium-high heat, cook bacon until crisp. Remove bacon with a slotted spoon to a paper towel. Pour fat from the skillet and return to heat. Crumble bacon onto paper towel, drain well, and return to the skillet. Add vinegar, honey, and lemon rind. Bring to boil.

3. Reduce heat and add potatoes, celery, parsley, salt, and pepper. Stir gently to mix well. Add apples and raisins. Heat mixture to just below boiling.

Tasty Tidbits _____

Serve this salad as a condiment for grilled meats or as a side for turkey at holiday feasts.

Baked Sweet Potato and Chili Sticks

Yields 8 cups fries
Prep time: 20 minutes
Cook time: 25–30 minutes
Serving size: 1 cup fries
Each serving:
Glycemic index: low
Glycemic load: 15
Calories: 225
Protein: 3 grams
Carbohydrates: 33 grams
Fiber: 6 grams
Fat: 9 grams
Saturated fat: 4 grams

Crunchy baked "fries" flavored with chili and dipped in sour cream-cilantro sauce.

5–6 (3.5 lbs.) large sweet potatoes, unpeeled

2 TB. olive oil

¾ tsp. salt

¼ tsp. freshly ground black pepper

½ cup orange juice

3½ tsp. chili powder

1 TB. honey

1 (8-oz.) pkg. dairy sour cream

⅓ cup fresh cilantro, chopped

1. Preheat the oven to 450°F.

2. Cut potatoes into 1-inch-thick wedges. Place in a large resealable plastic bag; add olive oil, salt, and pepper and toss.

3. Arrange potatoes in 2 (13×9×2-inch) baking pans.

4. In a small bowl, mix orange juice, 3 teaspoons of the chili powder, and honey.

5. Bake potato wedges, uncovered, for 25–30 minutes, or until tender, brushing 3 times with orange juice mixture and shaking pans occasionally.

6. In a second small bowl, mix sour cream, ½ teaspoon chili powder, and cilantro. Transfer potatoes to a serving dish. Serve with sour cream mixture for dipping.

Variation: Omit the sour cream dipping sauce and serve sweet potato sticks plain.

 Tasty Tidbits

Sweet potato sticks are a superb substitute for french fries. They're low glycemic, nutrient-dense, and baked, not fried. They taste terrific with or without sauce.

Sweet Potato Pancakes

Savory sweet potato cakes flavored with onion and parsley.

4 large sweet potatoes, uncooked

½ large onion, finely chopped

2 eggs, beaten

2 TB. flour

1 tsp. salt

½ tsp. baking soda

4 tsp. olive oil

Black pepper to taste

Yields 10 pancakes
Prep time: 20 minutes
Cook time: 10–15 minutes
Serving size: 2 pancakes
Each serving:
Glycemic index: low
Glycemic load: 17
Calories: 298
Protein: 5 grams
Carbohydrates: 38 grams
Fiber: 7 grams
Fat: 14 grams
Saturated fat: 2 grams

1. Finely shred potatoes. Grate onions. Place onion and potato in a large mixing bowl. Add eggs, flour, salt, and baking soda. Mix well. Mold mixture into pancakes 3-inches in diameter.

2. In a large skillet over medium-high heat, heat 2 teaspoons olive oil. Place 4–6 potato pancakes into a skillet and sauté until very well browned on one side. Turn once and brown on other side. Drain on paper towels. Sprinkle on black pepper.

3. Add any remaining pancakes to the pan with 2 tablespoons olive oil. Repeat cooking instructions in step 2.

4. These can be made in advance. They keep very well when frozen.

Variation: Omit onion and add 1 teaspoon cinnamon and ¼ teaspoon cloves for a sweet taste. Or season with ½ teaspoon chili powder and 2 tablespoon chopped fresh cilantro for a more savory taste.

Twice-Baked Sweet Potatoes

Cranberries, raisins, and walnuts enhance the potato flavor.

Yields 10 potato halves	

Prep time: 20 minutes

Cook time: 1 hour 40 minutes, plus 25–35 minutes

Serving size: ¹/₂ potato

Each serving:

Glycemic index: low

Glycemic load: 14

Calories: 195

Protein: 4 grams

Carbohydrates: 29 grams

Fiber: 4 grams

Fat: 7 grams

Saturated fat: 3 grams

5 (10-oz. ea.) medium-size sweet potatoes

¹/₂ cup cranberry relish

¹/₂ cup raisins, chopped

3 TB. butter, softened

¹/₂ tsp. salt

¹/₂ cup walnut pieces

1. Preheat the oven to 325°F.

2. Scrub sweet potatoes and pierce all over with a fork. Place on an oven rack. Bake for 1¹/₄ to 1¹/₂ hours until tender. Set aside to cool slightly.

3. Cut each potato in half lengthwise. Using a spoon, scoop pulp from each potato half, leaving a ¹/₄- to ¹/₂-inch shell. Place pulp in a medium-size bowl. Set aside shells.

4. Using a potato masher or a fork, mash potato pulp. Stir in cranberry relish, raisins, butter, and salt. Spoon potato mixture into each potato shell. Place, filled-sides up, in a 15×10×1-inch baking pan. Sprinkle each with walnut pieces.

5. Bake for 25–35 minutes until heated through.

 Home-Cooked Goodness

Tastes as sweet as candy, but these are a low-glycemic treat.

20

Fruit Side Dishes

In This Chapter

- ◆ Fruit makes an excellent side dish
- ◆ Lots of antioxidants and delightful colors
- ◆ Tangy, sweet, or spicy side dishes for variety

Fruit side dishes give you plenty of gustatory and health benefits. Fruit is naturally sweet and blends well with many spices to give you taste satisfaction and surprising accents to your main course.

Additionally, fruit contains concentrated antioxidants, vitamins, and minerals, making for a very nutritious addition to your low-glycemic meal. Indeed, fruit is the best way to satisfy your sweet tooth in a truly wholesome and varied way.

Baked Apples with Apricots

Yields 4 apples
Prep time: 15 minutes
Cook time: 45–60 minutes
Serving size: 1 apple
Each serving:
Glycemic index: low
Glycemic load: 15
Calories: 456
Protein: 8 grams
Carbohydrates: 52 grams
Fiber: 10 grams
Fat: 24 grams
Saturated fat: 5.1 grams

The almonds provide a nutty accent to the fruit flavor.

1 cup almonds, finely chopped

2 TB. butter, softened

1 tsp. honey

1 egg yolk

⅓ cup dried apricots, chopped

4 large cooking apples such as Granny Smith, Fuji, and Jonathan, about 8 oz. each

1. Preheat the oven to 400°F.

2. Beat together almonds, butter, honey, and egg yolk in a medium bowl. Stir in apricots.

3. Remove cores from apples using an apple corer, then cut a line with the point of a sharp knife around circumference of each apple.

4. Lightly grease a shallow baking dish. Arrange cooking apples in the dish.

5. Divide almond mixture among apples, filling the core of each. Bake for 45–60 minutes, until apples are soft.

Home-Cooked Goodness

Serve these apples cut in half and placed as a side dish with roast pork or chicken. You can even serve them for dessert.

Grapefruit and Avocado Salad

The grapefruit brings out the nutty taste of the avocados.

1 cup spinach, torn into bite-size pieces

3 cups romaine lettuce, torn into bite-size pieces

½ cup fresh cilantro, coarsely chopped

2 cups grapefruit, sectioned with membrane removed

2 medium avocados, halved, seeded, peeled, and cut into 1- to 2-inch pieces

2 TB. Parmesan cheese, shredded or shaved

Yields 4 salads
Prep time: 15 minutes
Cook time: none
Serving size: About 2 cups salad
Each serving:
Glycemic index: low
Glycemic load: 4
Calories: 179
Protein: 2 grams
Carbohydrates: 18 grams
Fiber: 2 grams
Fat: 11 grams
Saturated fat: 2 grams

1. Put spinach, romaine, and cilantro in a large salad bowl. Add grapefruit sections. Top with desired amount of Grapefruit and Olive Oil Dressing. See next recipe.

2. Divide onto 4 individual salad plates. On each plate, add ½ avocado and sprinkle with ½ tablespoon Parmesan cheese.

Grapefruit and Olive Oil Dressing

Grapefruit provides a tangy alternative to vinegar in this minty dressing.

¼ cup grapefruit juice

3 TB. olive oil

1 tsp. dried mint, crushed

½ tsp. freshly ground black pepper

¼ tsp. salt

Yields 1 cup salad dressing
Prep time: 5 minutes
Cook time: none
Serving size: 2 TB. salad dressing
Each serving:
Glycemic index: low
Glycemic load: <1
Calories: 63
Protein: 0 grams
Carbohydrates: 1 gram
Fiber: 0 grams
Fat: 1 gram
Saturated fat: 0 grams

Whisk together grapefruit juice, oil, mint, pepper, and salt.

Peach Salad with Thyme

If you love fresh peaches, you'll revel in the flavor combination of peaches, a savory dressing, pine nuts, and fresh thyme.

7 fresh, ripe medium-size peaches	**½ tsp. salt**
1½ cups water	**¼ tsp. ground black pepper**
2 sprigs fresh lemon thyme or thyme	**6 cups romaine lettuce, torn into bite-size pieces**
3 TB. lemon juice	**½ cup dried cranberries**
3 TB. honey	**¼ cup fresh chives, chopped**
2 TB. Dijon-style mustard	**¼ cup pine nuts, toasted**
⅓ cup olive oil	**2 tsp. fresh lemon thyme or thyme, chopped**

1. For dressing, halve and pit peaches. Coarsely chop 1 peach and set aside others. In a medium saucepan, combine chopped peach, water, and thyme sprigs. Bring to boil, then reduce heat. Simmer, uncovered, about 25 minutes or until liquid is reduced to ⅔ cup. Strain mixture and discard solids. Let syrup cool for 10 minutes.

2. Whisk in lemon juice, honey, and mustard to make dressing. Slowly whisk in oil, salt, and pepper. Set aside.

3. Slice remaining peaches. In a large salad bowl, combine sliced peaches, greens, cranberries, and chives. Toss with ¼ cup dressing. Divide salad among 6 salad plates. Sprinkle with pine nuts and chopped fresh thyme. Store remaining dressing in the refrigerator for up to 2 weeks.

Yields 12 cups salad

Prep time: 45 minutes

Cook time: 25 minutes, plus 10 minutes cool time

Serving size: 2 cups salad

Each serving:

Glycemic index: low

Glycemic load: 13

Calories: 290

Protein: 4 grams

Carbohydrates: 30 grams

Fiber: 5 grams

Fat: 17 grams

Saturated fat: 1 gram

Tasty Tidbits

Sometimes the word "salad" doesn't fit a recipe such as this. We think of it as fruit dressed up with salad greens. It tastes just as delicious, too.

Minted Melon and Berry Salad

This refreshing, simple-to-make minted salad's fresh, bright flavors will be a hit at family gatherings and picnics.

Yields 10 cups salad
Prep time: 15 minutes
Cook time: none
Serving size: 1 cup salad
Each serving:
Glycemic index: medium
Glycemic load: 14
Calories: 181
Protein: 1 gram
Carbohydrates: 24 grams
Fiber: 3 grams
Fat: 9 grams
Saturated fat: 1 gram

2 ripe honeydew melons, 2–2.5 pounds each

1 quart fresh strawberries, sliced (4.5 cups sliced)

2 TB. fresh mint, coarsely chopped

2 TB. raspberry vinegar

6 TB. olive oil

¼ tsp. salt

⅛ tsp. freshly ground black pepper

Fresh mint sprigs, to garnish

1. Halve melons, discarding seeds. Cut melons into 1-inch cubes or balls.

2. Wash, trim, and cut strawberries in half.

3. Place melon pieces and strawberries in a large serving bowl.

4. Make dressing by stirring mint, vinegar, oil, salt, and black pepper in a screw-top jar. Shake until blended.

5. Spoon mint dressing over melon and sliced strawberries. Garnish with mint sprig.

Variation: Substitute raspberries or blueberries for strawberries, and substitute cantaloupe for honeydew melon.

Home-Cooked Goodness

Ask the service personnel in your grocery store to select two ripe melons for you and ask how he or she determines ripeness. Eat within a day or two to enjoy melons at their peak of succulence.

Grilled Pineapple Salad

Yields 6 cups salad
Prep time: 20 minutes
Cook time: 5 minutes
Serving size: 1 cup salad
Each serving:
Glycemic index: low
Glycemic load: 15
Calories: 184
Protein: 1 gram
Carbohydrates: 30 grams
Fiber: 3 grams
Fat: 6.7 grams
Saturated fat: 1.6 grams

Tasty Tidbits

Grilling intensifies the flavor of fruit when the sugar contained within begins to caramelize. You can use an oven broiler to cook the fruit, if you prefer.

Grilled pineapple, mango, and nectarine are flavored with a creamy, tart-sweet dressing.

2 medium mangoes	**¼ cup yogurt, fat-free**
½ small pineapple (about 1 lb.)	**1 tsp. red wine vinegar**
	1 tsp. fresh lemon juice
2 nectarines	**2 tsp. sugar**
2 TB. olive oil	**4 TB. shredded coconut**

1. Heat a gas grill over medium-high heat. Oil the grill rack.

2. Stand mango on one of its narrow sides, with stem end facing you. Using a sharp knife, cut slices 1 inch thick on each side of pit. Remove peel from slices. Place slices in a bowl.

3. Cut pineapple into ½-inch pieces. Add to the bowl.

4. Cut nectarines in half and remove pit. Cut each half in half again and add to bowl. Drizzle fruit with 2 tablespoons olive oil and turn gently to coat evenly.

5. In a small bowl, whisk together yogurt, vinegar, and sugar. Set aside.

6. Arrange fruit in single layer in a grill basket. Place over hottest part of fire, turning once or twice, until surface of fruit begins to caramelize—about 5 minutes total.

7. Arrange fruit on a platter and drizzle with cream mixture. Top with shredded coconut.

Summer Fruit Skewers

Kiwi, peaches, and watermelon are accented with basil.

8–16 bamboo skewers

2 cups kiwi, thickly sliced

2 cups watermelon, cut into chunks

2 cups peach, cut into chunks

1 cup yogurt, plain, fat-free

¼ cup fresh basil, chopped

Yields 8 cups fruit + 1 bowl dip
Prep time: 30 minutes
Cook time: none
Serving size: 1 fruit wand
Each serving:
Glycemic index: low
Glycemic load: 16
Calories: 68
Protein: 1 gram
Carbohydrates: 16 grams
Fiber: 2 grams
Fat: 0 grams
Saturated fat: 0 grams

1. On each skewer, thread some kiwi, watermelon, and peach pieces. Place on a serving platter.

2. In a small serving bowl, stir together yogurt and basil. Serve fruit with sour cream dip.

Variation: Use lemon verbena or tarragon in place of basil.

Blueberries, Kiwi, and Spinach Salad

A spinach salad with fruit is accented with flavored vinegars.

6 kiwis

2 tsp. green onions, minced

3 tsp. balsamic vinegar

1 tsp. raspberry vinegar

2 tsp. olive oil

2 cups (8-oz.) blueberries

1 cup apricots, coarsely chopped

4 cups spinach leaves

¼ cup toasted slivered almonds

Yields 10 cups salad
Prep time: 20 minutes
Cook time: none
Serving size: 1¼ cup salad
Each serving:
Glycemic index: low
Glycemic load: 7
Calories: 116
Protein: 3 grams
Carbohydrates: 17 grams
Fiber: 4 grams
Fat: 4 grams
Saturated fat: <1 gram

1. Peel and slice kiwi. Set aside.

2. Put green onions in a salad bowl. Add balsamic and raspberry vinegars and olive oil. Whisk to blend.

3. Add blueberries, apricots, and spinach. Toss gently to coat. Add kiwi and almonds and toss again.

Green Salad with Apricot Vinaigrette

A leafy green salad is flavored with pears and oranges.

Yields 12 cups salad with vinaigrette
Prep time: 15 minutes
Cook time: none
Serving size: 2 cups salad with vinaigrette
Each serving:
Glycemic index: low
Glycemic load: 9
Calories: 205
Protein: 1 gram
Carbohydrates: 21 grams
Fiber: 3 grams
Fat: 13 grams
Saturated fat: 1 gram

¼ cup olive oil

¼ cup red-wine vinegar

2 TB. lemon juice

2 TB. apricot jam

⅛ tsp. red pepper flakes

2 ripe, firm, large pears, cored, and sliced

8 cups green and red leaf lettuce

1 (11-oz.) can unsweetened mandarin oranges, drained

¼ cup pecans, chopped

1. In a medium mixing bowl, whisk olive oil, red wine vinegar, lemon juice, apricot jam, and red pepper flakes. Add sliced pears and toss gently, coating pears to prevent browning.

2. In a large salad bowl, combine lettuce, oranges, and pecans. Add pear mixture to the bowl and toss gently.

Home-Cooked Goodness

Canned unsweetened mandarin oranges offer convenience when you can't find the time to peel, seed, and remove the membrane from oranges.

Red Salad with Honey Vinaigrette

Grapes, pomegranate, grapefruit, and Romaine flavored with toasted sunflower seeds for a nutty citrus taste.

⅓ cup olive oil

¼ cup orange juice

¼ cup balsamic vinegar

2 tsp. honey

¼ tsp. ground black pepper

8 cups red leaf lettuce

3 medium red or pink grapefruits

1½ cups red seedless grapes

4 TB. pomegranate seeds

3 TB. salted toasted sunflower seeds

Yields 12 cups salad with vinaigrette
Prep time: 25 minutes
Cook time: none
Serving size: 1 cup salad with vinaigrette
Each serving:
Glycemic index: low
Glycemic load: 6
Calories: 217
Protein: 3 grams
Carbohydrates: 22 grams
Fiber: 3 grams
Fat: 13 grams
Saturated fat: 1 gram

1. For dressing, whisk together olive oil, orange juice, balsamic vinegar, honey, and black pepper in a small bowl.

2. Peel and section grapefruits. Place in a side bowl.

3. In a large salad bowl, place lettuce, grapefruit sections, grapes, and pomegranate seeds. Toss with dressing. Sprinkle with sunflower seeds.

Home-Cooked Goodness

A salad with red fruits, such as this one, is full of healthy antioxidants—you can tell by the bright colors.

Fruit with Rosemary

A simple but elegant citrus salad flavored with fresh rosemary.

3 large grapefruit	**1 tsp. fresh rosemary, chopped**
3 medium oranges	

Yields 8 cups fruit
Prep time: 20 minutes
Cook time: none
Serving size: 1¹/₃ cups fruit
Each serving:
Glycemic index: low
Glycemic load: 7
Calories: 100
Protein: 2 grams
Carbohydrates: 23 grams
Fiber: 3 grams
Fat: 0 grams
Saturated fat: 0 grams

1. Using a sharp paring knife, peel skin and outer pulp from grapefruit and oranges. Slice from outside toward center, along each side of the membranes, to remove whole fruit sections. Discard seeds.

2. Arrange alternate sections of grapefruit and oranges in a windmill effect on a serving platter. Sprinkle with rosemary.

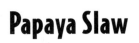

Papaya Slaw

Spicy papaya seeds and sweet papaya fruit flavor this cabbage and cilantro slaw.

¼ cup mayonnaise	**4 cups (6-oz.) coleslaw mix**
2 TB. lemon juice	**1 ripe papaya (about 1 lb.), peeled and coarsely diced, reserve seeds**
1 TB. red wine vinegar	
½ tsp. salt	**1 small red bell pepper, sliced**
½ tsp. freshly ground black pepper	**½ cup fresh cilantro, chopped**

Yields 7 cups slaw
Prep time: 20 minutes
Cook time: none
Serving size: 1³/₄ cups slaw
Each serving:
Glycemic index: low
Glycemic load: 8
Calories: 200
Protein: 3 grams
Carbohydrates: 20 grams
Fiber: 4 grams
Fat: 12 grams
Saturated fat: 1 gram

1. In a small bowl, whisk together mayonnaise, lemon juice, vinegar, salt, and pepper.

2. In a salad bowl, place coleslaw mix, papaya, red bell pepper, and cilantro. Toss with mayonnaise mixture. Top with papaya seeds.

Strawberry Salad with Cinnamon

Salad greens with strawberries and avocado are made sweet and spicy with hot pepper sauce and strawberry jam.

3 TB. olive oil

3 TB. cup raspberry vinegar

1 TB. strawberry jam or jelly

¼ tsp. hot pepper sauce

¼ tsp. salt

⅛ tsp. freshly ground black pepper

¼ tsp. cinnamon

12 cups romaine, torn into bite-size pieces

1 pint strawberries, stemmed and quartered

½ small red onion, peeled and thinly sliced

½ cup pecans, coarsely chopped

1 avocado, about 4 oz., peeled, seeded, and sliced

Yields 16 cups salad with dressing	
Prep time: 20 minutes	
Cook time: none	
Serving size: 2 cups salad with dressing	
Each serving:	
Glycemic index: low	
Glycemic load: 2	
Calories: 157	
Protein: 2 grams	
Carbohydrates: 8 grams	
Fiber: 3 grams	
Fat: 13 grams	
Saturated fat: 1 gram	

1. For dressing, whisk oil, vinegar, jam or jelly, hot pepper sauce, salt, pepper, and cinnamon in a small bowl.

2. In a salad bowl, combine lettuce, strawberries, red onion, pecans, and avocado. Toss with dressing.

Home-Cooked Goodness

The strawberry jam strengthens the strawberry flavor and adds very few calories with virtually no increase in glycemic value.

Curried Waldorf Salad with Dates

Yields 8 cups salad
Prep time: 20 minutes
Cook time: none
Serving size: 1 cup salad
Each serving:
Glycemic index: low
Glycemic load: 7
Calories: 210
Protein: 3 grams
Carbohydrates: 18 grams
Fiber: 3 grams
Fat: 14 grams
Saturated fat: 3 grams

Apples and celery wrapped in a tangy mayonnaise dressing, spiced up with curry and red pepper, and accented with walnuts and dates.

⅓ cup mayonnaise

¼ cup sour cream

1 TB. fresh lemon juice

1 tsp. honey

½ tsp. salt

½ tsp. ground curry

⅛ tsp. red pepper flakes

3 large red apples (about 8 oz.), cored, cut into ⅜-inch pieces

3 ribs celery, cut lengthwise in half, then sliced into ⅜-inch slices

½ cup walnuts, coarsely chopped

⅓ cup dates, coarsely chopped

1. In a small bowl, whisk together mayonnaise, sour cream, lemon juice, honey, salt, curry, and red pepper.

2. In a mixing bowl, place apples, celery, walnuts, and dates. Toss with desired amount of mayonnaise mixture.

Home-Cooked Goodness

Red pepper and curry add a flavor surprise to the traditional Waldorf salad. Serve it as a side with main dish salads and brunch. It's also delicious for dessert.

Chapter 21

Grains

In This Chapter

- ◆ A wide variety of grains
- ◆ Low-glycemic with a higher-glycemic load
- ◆ Fun grain-and-vegetable combinations

Most unrefined grains are low-glycemic, though not low in carbohydrates. They work well as side dishes in a glycemic index eating program.

In this chapter you'll find varied recipes for barley, corn meal, many types of rice, quinoa, and wheat berries. You'll enjoy the crunchy and distinct flavors of these grains and the interesting pairings with vegetables, fruit, nuts, herbs, and spices.

Wild Rice Pilaf with Vegetables

Cranberries and thyme add flavor to the rice and vegetables.

1 cup uncooked wild rice (3 cups cooked)	**½ fennel bulb (8-oz.), trimmed and chopped**
¼ tsp. salt	**1 medium onion, chopped**
2 cups water	**2 TB. butter**
¾ cup dried cranberries	**¼ tsp. dried thyme**
3 carrots, peeled and chopped	**½ tsp. salt**
1 rib celery, chopped	**¼ tsp. freshly ground black pepper**

1. Rinse wild rice. In a large saucepan over high heat, bring wild rice, salt, and water to boil. Reduce heat. Cover and simmer for 45–60 minutes. Stir in dried cranberries. Drain, if necessary.

2. In another large saucepan fitted with a vegetable steamer, add carrots, celery, fennel, and onion. Cook until vegetables are tender—about 5–10 minutes. Place in serving bowl. Stir in butter cut into small pieces and thyme. Sprinkle with salt and pepper. Add wild rice to vegetables. Stir and serve.

Yields 8 cups pilaf
Prep time: 20 minutes
Cook time: 65–85 minutes
Serving size: 1 cup pilaf
Each serving:
Glycemic index: low
Glycemic load: 16
Calories: 167
Protein: 5 grams
Carbohydrates: 30 grams
Fiber: 3 grams
Fat: 3 grams
Saturated fat: 1.75 grams

Greek Rice Pilaf

Brown rice with the subtle flavors of oregano and lemon.

2 TB. butter	**2 cups water**
2 cups brown rice (4 cups cooked)	**2 cups natural chicken broth**
3 TB. fresh lemon juice	**¼ tsp. oregano**
	½ cup fresh tomato, diced

1. In a medium saucepan over medium heat, melt butter. Sauté brown rice for 2–3 minutes. Pour lemon juice over rice and simmer for 2 minutes.

2. Pour water and broth into the saucepan. Increase heat to high and bring to boil. Stir well. Cover and simmer over low heat for 20 minutes or until rice is just tender. Stir in oregano and tomato.

Yields 4½ cups pilaf
Prep time: 15 minutes
Cook time: 25 minutes
Serving size: ½ cup pilaf
Each serving:
Glycemic index: low
Glycemic load: 11
Calories: 119
Protein: 3 grams
Carbohydrates: 20 grams
Fiber: 2 grams
Fat: 3 grams
Saturated fat: 1.5 grams

Chilled Rice Salad with Ham

Soy sauce and raisins enhance this rice and ham side salad.

3 cups cooked basmati rice, cooled

1 cup low-fat 5 percent ham, diced

¼ cup green onion, diced

1 cup green or red bell peppers, diced

¼ cup golden raisins

½ cup mayonnaise

2 TB. soy sauce

¼ tsp. salt

⅛ tsp. freshly ground black pepper

Yields 6 cups salad
Prep time: 15 minutes
Cook time: none
Serving size: 1 cup salad
Each serving:
Glycemic index: medium
Glycemic load: 16
Calories: 301
Protein: 12 grams
Carbohydrates: 28 grams
Fiber: 3 grams
Fat: 15.7 grams
Saturated fat: 2.6 grams

1. In a large mixing bowl, combine rice, ham, onion, peppers, and raisins.

2. In a small bowl, whisk together mayonnaise, soy sauce, salt, and pepper. Pour over rice mixture and mix well. Chill at least 1 hour before serving.

Tabbouleh with Tomatoes and Mint

A Middle Eastern favorite flavored with mint and lemon.

1½ cups bulgur wheat

¼ cup fresh lemon juice

1½ cups boiling water

3 medium ripe tomatoes, coarsely diced

1 medium cucumber, cut into ½-inch slices

3 green onions, chopped

½ tsp. minced garlic

¾ cup parsley, chopped

½ cup mint leaves, chopped

1 TB. olive oil

¾ tsp. salt

¼ tsp. freshly ground black pepper

¼ tsp. crushed red pepper

Yields 8 cups tabbouleh
Prep time: 30 minutes, plus 30 minutes chill time
Cook time: none
Serving size: 1 cup tabbouleh
Each serving:
Glycemic index: low
Glycemic load: 7
Calories: 128
Protein: 4 grams
Carbohydrates: 19 grams
Fiber: 5 grams
Fat: 4 grams
Saturated fat: <1 gram

1. In a medium bowl, combine bulgur, lemon juice, and boiling water. Let stand 30 minutes, or until liquid is absorbed.

2. Add tomatoes, cucumber, green onions, garlic, parsley, mint, oil, salt, black pepper, and crushed pepper. Stir to mix. Cover and refrigerate at least 30 minutes before serving.

Risotto Italiano

A robust vegetable and rice dish flavored with parsley and garlic.

Yields about 8 cups risotto
Prep time: 15 minutes
Cook time: 25 minutes
Serving size: 1 cup risotto
Each serving:
Glycemic index: low
Glycemic load: 10
Calories: 118
Protein: 5 grams
Carbohydrates: 22 grams
Fiber: 4 grams
Fat: 6 grams
Saturated fat: 2.25 grams

2 TB. butter

½ cup onion, chopped

½ tsp. minced garlic

1 cup uncooked basmati rice

3 cups natural chicken stock

1 TB. olive oil

¾ cup fresh tomatoes, chopped

1 (14-oz.) can artichokes

½ cup carrots, julienned

½ cup zucchini, julienned

½ cup fresh green beans

1 (2.25-oz.) can sliced black olives

¼ cup dry white wine

¼ cup Parmesan cheese, freshly grated

¼ cup fresh parsley, chopped

½ tsp. salt

¼ tsp. freshly ground black pepper

1 inch anchovy paste (optional)

Tasty Tidbits

Purchase anchovy paste and keep on hand to flavor salad dressings and Italian dishes like this risotto. Just a little adds a savory, authentic taste.

1. Heat butter in a medium saucepan over medium-low heat. Add onion and garlic and cook until translucent. Add rice. Sauté for 5 minutes, or until rice is lightly toasted, stirring constantly.

2. Heat chicken stock in a medium saucepan over medium-high heat. Stir in rice. Cover and cook over medium-low heat until broth is absorbed—about 20 minutes.

3. In a medium skillet over medium-high heat, combine olive oil, tomatoes, artichokes, carrots, zucchini, green beans, and olives. Sauté vegetables for 5 minutes.

4. Stir in rice, wine, Parmesan, parsley, salt, pepper, and anchovy paste (if using).

Lemon and Parsley Risotto Cake

Asiago and mozzarella cheeses add flavor to this risotto, accented with parsley and chives.

1¼ cups long-grain white rice

2½ cups water

1 lemon rind, finely grated

2 TB. fresh chives, chopped

2 TB. fresh parsley, chopped

¼ cup part skim milk mozza-rella cheese, grated

¼ cup Asiago cheese, grated

½ tsp. salt

¼ tsp. freshly ground black pepper

Yields 1 (9×5×3-inch) pan
Prep time: 15 minutes
Cook time: 55 minutes
Serving size: 1 slice cake
Each serving:
Glycemic index: medium
Glycemic load: 9
Calories: 103
Protein: 5 grams
Carbohydrates: 14 grams
Fiber: <1 gram
Fat: 3 grams
Saturated fat: 2 grams

1. Preheat the oven to 400°F.

2. In a medium skillet, add rice and water.

3. Bring to boil. Cover pan and simmer gently, stirring occasionally, for about 20 minutes, or until liquid is absorbed.

4. Stir in lemon rind, chives, parsley, mozzarella, Asiago, salt, and pepper.

5. Spoon into a 9×5×3-inch loaf pan, cover with foil, and bake for 30–35 minutes or until lightly browned. Turn out and serve in slices.

Home-Cooked Goodness

This recipe calls for a low-glycemic rice rather than the traditional sticky risotto rice. The rice mixture is held together by the baked cheeses.

Polenta with Rosemary

Italian-style polenta is accented with Parmesan and rosemary.

Yields 4–5 cups polenta
Prep time: 30 minutes
Cook time: 15 minutes
Serving size: ¹/₂ cup polenta
Each serving:
Glycemic index: medium
Glycemic load: 10
Calories: 108
Protein: 3 grams
Carbohydrates: 15 g
Fiber: 2 g
Fat: 4 g
Saturated fat: 2 grams

1 cup cold water

½ tsp. salt

¾ cup coarse cornmeal

2¼ cups boiling water

¼ cup Parmesan, freshly grated

2 TB. butter

¼ tsp. dried rosemary

1. In a large saucepan, combine cold water and salt. With wire whisk, gradually beat in cornmeal until smooth. Whisk in boiling water.

2. Heat to boiling over high heat. Reduce heat to medium-low and cook, stirring frequently with a wooden spoon until mixture is very thick, for 20–25 minutes.

3. Stir Parmesan, butter, and rosemary into polenta until butter is melted. Serve immediately.

Home-Cooked Goodness

Save leftovers in the refrigerator in a glass food-storage dish. Use glass because you can safely reheat in it and glass preserves the delicious taste clearly without adding a faint plastic-type odor. Slice polenta and sauté for breakfast. Serve with sausage or bacon and eggs and fruit.

Quinoa Salad with Green Chiles

The nutty flavor of quinoa is combined with garlic, green chile, and pinion nuts.

4 (4-oz.) cans whole green chiles, mild or jalapeño

2 cups quinoa

2 cups water

1 cup green onions, chopped

2 TB. butter

⅓ cup olive oil

⅓ cup lime juice

4 tsp. minced garlic

½ tsp. salt

¼ tsp. freshly ground black pepper

2 cups fresh cilantro, lightly chopped

⅔ cup pine nuts

8 leaves Bibb lettuce

1. Preheat the oven to 425°F.

2. Halve chile peppers lengthwise. Cut peppers in bite-size strips. Set aside.

3. In a colander, rinse quinoa in cold water. In a medium saucepan over high heat, combine quinoa and water. Bring to boil. Reduce heat to medium-low and simmer, covered, for 25 minutes. Remove from heat. Uncover. Let stand about 30 minutes.

4. Meanwhile, in a medium skillet over medium heat, sauté green onions in butter until tender. Remove from heat. Cool.

5. For vinaigrette, combine olive oil, lime juice, garlic, sea salt, and black pepper in a small screw-top jar. Cover and shake well to combine.

6. In a mixing bowl, combine quinoa, chile pepper strips, green onions, vinaigrette, cilantro, and pine nuts.

7. Line a platter with lettuce. Top with salad. Serve at room temperature.

Yields 8 cups salad
Prep time: 20 minutes
Cook time: 25 minutes, plus 30 minutes stand time
Serving size: 1 cup salad
Each serving:
Glycemic index: low
Glycemic load: 17
Calories: 273
Protein: 6 grams
Carbohydrates: 33 grams
Fiber: 4 grams
Fat: 13 grams
Saturated fat: 3 grams

Home-Cooked Goodness

Quinoa has a low glycemic index value of 53 with a high carbohydrate count, so enjoy, but eat sparingly. It originated in the Andes Mountains of South America. Combine with vegetables to increase your daily vegetable intake.

Wheat Berries with Pecans

Mushrooms sautéed in butter and the accent of pecans add festive flavor to wheat berries.

Yields 6 cups wheat berries

Prep time: 15 minutes, plus soak overnight

Cook time: 1 hour 20 minutes

Serving size: ³/₄ cup wheat berries

Each serving:

Glycemic index: low

Glycemic load: 9

Calories: 218

Protein: 7 grams

Carbohydrates: 25 grams

Fiber: 5 grams

Fat: 10 grams

Saturated fat: 3 grams

1 cup wheat berries	½ cup pecans
3 cups water	½ tsp. salt
2 TB. butter	¼ tsp. freshly ground black pepper
1 green onion, chopped	
4 cups mushrooms, sliced	

1. In mixing bowl, soak wheat berries overnight in just enough water to cover them. The next morning, drain.

2. In a large saucepan over high heat, bring water and wheat berries to boil. Reduce heat. Cover and simmer until berries are tender but firm—about 1 hour. Drain.

3. In a large skillet over medium heat, sauté butter and green onions for 2 minutes. Add mushrooms and sauté until tender—about 6–10 minutes. Stir in pecans, salt, and pepper and cook, stirring, for 5 minutes.

4. Add wheat berries to the saucepan. Stir and heat thoroughly.

Home-Cooked Goodness

Purchase wheat berries at the health food section of your local grocery, or at a health food store. Serve with hearty pot roasts and stews.

Barley and Nectarine Salad

Basil adds fresh flavor to this mixed grain and fruit salad.

3 cups water

½ (16-oz.) package pearl barley

2½ tsp. salt

1 TB. lime peel

¼ cup fresh lime juice

¼ cup olive oil

1 TB. honey

½ tsp. freshly ground black pepper

2 medium nectarines, cut into ½-inch pieces

1 large tomato, cut into ½-inch pieces

1 green onion, thinly sliced

¼ cup fresh basil, chopped

Yields 8 cups salad
Prep time: 30 minutes
Cook time: 55 minutes
Serving size: 1 cup salad
Each serving:
Glycemic index: low
Glycemic load: 7
Calories: 191
Protein: 3 grams
Carbohydrates: 29 grams
Fiber: 5 grams
Fat: 7 grams
Saturated fat: 1 gram

1. In a large saucepan over high heat, boil water. Add barley and 1½ teaspoon salt. Reduce heat. Cover and simmer about 45 minutes, until water is absorbed and barley is tender.

2. In a large bowl, whisk together lime peel, lime juice, oil, honey, 1 teaspoon salt, and pepper.

3. Rinse barley and drain. Add barley, nectarines, tomatoes, green onions, and basil to dressing. Stir gently to mix.

Tasty Tidbits _____

Grow fresh basil in your garden and use it to flavor your meals throughout the summer. In autumn, harvest leaves, wash, dry, and freeze in food-storage bags to use during the winter and early spring.

Part 6

Sweet Endings

Go ahead, satisfy your sweet tooth with these lower-glycemic recipes. Our fruit desserts give you at least one serving of fruit with a sweetness that finishes your meal. Dig into our pies, cakes, cookies, and puddings lightly. Savor each bite and think of eating tastes, certainly not platefuls.

If chocolate is one of the great loves of your life, you'll delight in our recipes for brownies, cakes, mousses, and more.

Our beverage chapter solves a challenging problem: what beverages are both low glycemic and healthful? You'll find lemonades, teas, fruit punches, hot cocoa, and more

Chapter 22

Fruit Desserts

In This Chapter

- Light tastes for satisfying desserts
- Using honey with fruit
- Spices and herbs that accent fresh fruit

Fruit is wonderful for dessert. Savor each bite of delicious fruit, knowing that you're eating at least one more healthful serving of fruit to support your daily intake of 5–10 servings of vegetables and fruit.

We classified a fruit dish as a dessert if the recipe included added sweetener. Most of the recipes in this chapter call for a bit of honey, while some use sugar. Our fruit desserts also don't call for flour or other baking ingredients—we've saved baking recipes for our other two dessert chapters—Chapters 23 and 24.

Yields 2 cups fruit and 1 dip

Prep time: 15 minutes

Cook time: none

Serving size: ¹/₂ cup fruit and ¹/₄ dip

Each serving (¹/₂ cup straw-berries):

Glycemic index: low

Glycemic load: 2

Calories: 26

Protein: <1 gram

Carbohydrates: 6 grams

Fiber: 2 grams

Fat: 0 grams

Saturated fat: 0 grams

Each serving (¹/₂ cup white grapes):

Glycemic index: low

Glycemic load: 7

Calories: 60

Protein: <1 gram

Carbohydrates: 15 grams

Fiber: 1 gram

Fat: 0 grams

Saturated fat: 0 grams

Each serving (¹/₂ cup apples):

Glycemic index: low

Glycemic load: 4

Calories: 45

Protein: <1 gram

Carbohydrates: 11 grams

Fiber: 2 grams

Fat: 0 grams

Saturated fat: 0 grams

Each serving (¹/₂ cup fresh pineapple):

Glycemic index: medium

Glycemic load: 7

Calories: 45

Protein: <1 gram

Carbohydrates: 11 grams

Fiber: 1 gram

Fat: 0 grams

Saturated fat: 0 grams

Each serving (¹/₂ cup black grapes):

Glycemic index: medium

Glycemic load: 9

Calories: 60

Protein: <1 gram

Carbohydrates: 15 grams

Fiber: 1 gram

Fat: 0 grams

Saturated fat: 0 grams

Each serving (¹/₂ cup fresh pears):

Glycemic index: low

Glycemic load: 4

Calories: 45

Protein: <1 gram

Carbohydrates: 11 grams

Fiber: 2 grams

Fat: 0 grams

Saturated fat: 0 grams

Each serving (¹/₂ cup fresh peaches):

Glycemic index: low

Glycemic load: 3

Calories: 30

Protein: <1 gram

Carbohydrates: 7 grams

Fiber: 1 gram

Fat: 0 grams

Saturated fat: 0 grams

Fresh Fruit Fondue

You have your pick of flavors: sour cream and brown sugar, chocolate and nuts, honey and pepper, cinnamon, or sesame.

2 cups fruit for dipping (strawberries, pineapple pieces, grapes, peach or nectarine wedges, orange sections, apple or pear wedges.

Two dips (choose from the following recipes)

Long toothpicks to hold fruit for dipping

See directions for eating below.

Sour Cream and Sugar Dip

¼ **cup sour cream**

2 TB. brown sugar

Place sour cream in a small bowl, and brown sugar in another bowl. Place fruit on toothpicks. Dip each piece of fruit first in sour cream and next in brown sugar. Then eat.

Yields 1 dip
Prep time: 5 minutes
Cook time: none
Serving size: 1½ TB.
Each serving:
Glycemic index: medium
Glycemic load: 7
Calories: 76
Protein: <1 gram
Carbohydrates: 10 grams
Fiber: 0 grams
Fat: 4 grams
Saturated fat: 2.3 grams

Chocolate and Nuts Dip

Yields 1 dip	
Prep time: 10 minutes	
Cook time: none	
Serving size: 2 TB.	
Each serving:	
Glycemic index: low	
Glycemic load: 6	
Calories: 127	
Protein: 1 gram	
Carbohydrates: 15 grams	
Fiber: 0 grams	
Fat: 8 grams	
Saturated fat: 2 grams	

6 oz. milk chocolate morsels or bars (12 TB.)   **¼ cup salted nuts, chopped (4 TB.)**

1. Melt chocolate in a small saucepan. Spoon into a small bowl.

2. Place nuts in another small bowl. Dip fruit first in chocolate, then in nuts.

Honey Pepper Dip

Yields 1 dip	
Prep time: 5 minutes	
Cook time: none	
Serving size: 1¹/₂ TB.	
Each serving:	
Glycemic index: low	
Glycemic load: 10	
Calories: 88	
Protein: 0 grams	
Carbohydrates: 22 grams	
Fiber: 0 grams	
Fat: 0 grams	
Saturated fat: 0 grams	

¼ cup honey   **2 TB. cracked black pepper or paprika**

Set out one bowl with honey, and one with pepper or paprika. Dip fruit into honey and then into pepper or paprika.

Cinnamon Sour Cream Dip

1 tsp. cinnamon   ¼ cup sour cream

Stir cinnamon into sour cream. Spoon into a serving bowl. Dip fruit and enjoy.

Yields 1 dip
Prep time: 5 minutes
Cook time: none
Serving size: 1 TB. dip
Each serving has:
Glycemic index: very low
Glycemic load: 0
Calories: 23
Protein: <1 gram
Carbohydrates: <1 gram
Fiber: 0 grams
Fat: 2.5 grams
Saturated fat: 1.6 grams

Sesame Seed Honey Dip

¼ cup honey   4 TB. sesame seeds

Place honey in one bowl and sesame seeds in another bowl. Dip fruit into honey, then into sesame seeds.

Tasty Tidbits

The activity of eating fondue creates an atmosphere of fun and intimacy. Share with family and friends for special celebrations.

Yields 1 dip
Prep time: 5 minutes
Cook time: none
Serving size: 2 TB. dip
Each serving:
Glycemic index: low
Glycemic load: 16
Calories: 200
Protein: <1 gram
Carbohydrates: 30 grams
Fiber: 1 gram
Fat: 8.9 grams
Saturated fat: 1.3 grams

Oranges in Cinnamon Caramel Sauce

An interesting combination of oranges and cinnamon, sweetened with burnt sugar caramel.

Yields 8 oranges
Prep time: 20 minutes
Cook time: 10 minutes
Serving size: 1 orange and 1½ tsp. pistachios and pomegranate seeds
Each serving:
Glycemic index: low
Glycemic load: 13
Calories: 126
Protein: 2 grams
Carbohydrates: 25 grams
Fiber: 3 grams
Fat: 2 grams
Saturated fat: <1 gram

8 clementines, tangerines, or other small, easily-peeled oranges

½ cup sugar

1½ cups warm water

2 cinnamon sticks

¼ cup pomegranate seeds

¼ cup shelled pistachio nuts

1. Pare rind from two clementines, tangerines, or oranges using a vegetable peeler, and cut into fine strips. Set aside.

2. Peel oranges and separate the sections. Place in a serving bowl.

3. In a saucepan over medium heat, stir sugar until dissolved and becomes a rich golden brown color. Remove the saucepan from heat.

4. Slowly pour water into the saucepan. Be careful—the water may splatter. Return the saucepan to medium-high heat and bring slowly to a boil, stirring until caramel dissolves. Lower heat to medium-low. Add shredded peel and cinnamon sticks. Simmer for 5 minutes.

5. Cool syrup for about 10 minutes. Pour over oranges. Cover the serving bowl and chill for several hours or overnight.

6. To serve, place orange sections on individual plates and sprinkle with pomegranate seeds and pistachios.

 Tasty Tidbits

Because oranges are plentiful in all seasons, you can enjoy this dessert year-round. Substitute raspberries or blueberries for pomegranate seeds, if you like.

Baked Pears

Baked pears given a rich, caramel flavor by rum and almonds.

¼ cup lime juice

¼ cup honey

⅓ cup light rum

4 large pears, peeled, halved, and cored

¼ cup slivered almonds

¼ cup sour cream

Yields 4 pears
Prep time: 15 minutes
Bake time: 1 hour
Serving size: ½ pear
Each serving:
Glycemic index: low
Glycemic load: 9
Calories: 127
Protein: 2 grams
Carbohydrates: 23 grams
Fiber: 2 grams
Fat: 3 grams
Saturated fat: 1 gram

1. Preheat the oven to 325°F.

2. In a small bowl, whisk together lime juice, honey, and rum. Place pears in a 9×13-inch glass baking dish. Spoon some lime juice mixture into cavity of each pear half.

3. Bake 1 hour, basting frequently with remaining rum mixture, until pears are tender.

4. Sprinkle with almonds. Serve with sour cream.

Fresh Figs with Coffee

Coffee turns up the flavor of the figs and honey.

12 firm fresh figs

1½ cups freshly brewed coffee

⅓ cup honey

1 tsp. vanilla extract

Yields 24 fig halves
Prep time: 10 minutes
Cook time: 10 minutes
Serving size: 3 fig halves
Each serving:
Glycemic index: medium
Glycemic load: 15
Calories: 108
Protein: 1 gram
Carbohydrates: 26 grams
Fiber: 2 grams
Fat: <1 gram
Saturated fat: 0 grams

1. Pierce skin of figs with a fork in several places. Cut figs in half.

2. In a large skillet over high heat, combine coffee, honey, and vanilla extract. Cook until reduced to about ³/₄ cup.

3. Add figs to syrup, reduce heat, then cover and simmer for 5 minutes. Remove from heat. Serve at room temperature.

Figs in Ginger Sauce

Yields 6 cups figs in sauce
Prep time: 15 minutes
Cook time: 30–40 minutes
Serving size: ³/₄ cup figs in sauce
Each serving:
Glycemic index: medium
Glycemic load: 26
Calories: 221
Protein: 2 grams
Carbohydrates: 42 grams
Fiber: 6 grams
Fat: 5 grams
Saturated fat: 4 grams

Figs are festive when flavored with ginger and lemon.

1 lb. dried figs

2 cups water

3 TB. fresh lemon juice

1 TB. finely sliced lemon rind

1 (2-inch) piece ginger root, peeled, sliced in 4 pieces

¼ cup sugar

4 lemon slices

½ cup heavy cream

1. Wash figs and clip off stems. Place in a medium saucepan and add cold water to cover. Stir in 2 tablespoon lemon juice and lemon rind.

2. Add ginger root and bring mixture to a boil over high heat. Reduce heat to a slow boil. Cook until figs are puffed and soft—about 20–30 minutes. With a slotted spoon, remove figs to a serving dish.

3. Add sugar and simmer with 1 tablespoon lemon juice and 4 slices of lemon.

4. Pour syrup over figs. Chill and serve with cream.

Glycemic Notes

Cook the figs until they are puffy and soft. Be careful. If you cook too long, they'll become mushy.

Fresh Sweet Cherry Bowl

The cherries are accented with sour cream cheese sauce.

½ cup sour cream

1 (3-oz.) pkg. cream cheese

3 TB. powdered sugar

1 TB. cherry brandy, cider, or juice

3½ cups fresh Rainier or Bing cherries, pitted

½ cup slivered almonds

Yields 5 cups sauce
Prep time: 20 minutes
Cook time: none
Serving size: ¹/₂ cup sauce
Each serving:
Glycemic index: low
Glycemic load: 6
Calories: 122
Protein: 1 gram
Carbohydrates: 16 grams
Fiber: 2 grams
Fat: 6 grams
Saturated fat: 3 grams

1. In a medium mixing bowl, combine sour cream, cream cheese, powdered sugar, and liqueur or cider. Beat with an electric mixer on low speed until smooth.

2. Divide cherries among 8 individual serving dishes. Top with sour cream mixture and sprinkle with almonds.

Bananas with Rum and Raisins

Bananas are spiced up with raisins, pecans, and cinnamon.

¼ cup raisins

4 TB. dark rum

2 TB. butter

¼ cup light brown sugar

4 bananas, peeled and halved lengthwise

¼ tsp. grated nutmeg

¼ tsp. ground cinnamon

2 TB. pecans, toasted and coarsely chopped

8 (¼-cup) scoops natural vanilla ice cream

Yields 8 bananas and 1 cup sauce
Prep time: 10 minutes
Cook time: 10 minutes
Serving size: 1 banana, ¹/₄ cup ice cream, 2 TB. sauce
Each serving:
Glycemic index: low
Glycemic load: 16
Calories: 141
Protein: 2 grams
Carbohydrates: 22 grams
Fiber: 1 gram
Fat: 5 grams
Saturated fat: 4 grams

1. Place raisins in a small bowl, cover with rum, and soak for about 30 minutes.

2. Melt butter in a skillet, add sugar, and stir until dissolved. Add raisins and bananas and cook for 2–3 minutes.

3. Sprinkle nutmeg and cinnamon over bananas. Remove to a serving dish. Sprinkle with pecans.

4. Serve immediately with single scoop of ice cream.

Thai Bananas

Bananas have an exotic taste with brown sugar and toasted coconut.

Yields 4 bananas and sauce
Prep time: 10 minutes
Cook time: 10 minutes
Serving size: ¹/₂ banana and ¹/₈ sauce, and ¹/₂ cup yogurt
Each serving:
Glycemic index: medium
Glycemic load: 13
Calories: 165
Protein: 6 grams
Carbohydrates: 24 grams
Fiber: 1 gram
Fat: 5 grams
Saturated fat: 3 grams

4 large slightly underripe bananas

3 TB. butter

1 TB. dried shredded coconut

4 TB. brown sugar

4 TB. lime juice

½ cup plain yogurt

1. Peel bananas and cut in half lengthwise. Heat butter in a large skillet and sauté bananas for 1–2 minutes on each side, until they are lightly golden in color.

2. In a small skillet over medium-high heat, sauté coconut, stirring often, until lightly browned—about 5 minutes.

3. Sprinkle brown sugar on bananas. Add lime juice and cook, stirring, until brown sugar is dissolved. Remove bananas and sauce to a serving bowl. Sprinkle coconut over bananas and serve with yogurt.

Summer Fruit with Minted Honey

Luscious fruit flavored with minted honey and lime juice.

Yields 8 cups fruit
Prep time: 20 minutes
Serving size: 1 cup fruit
Each serving:
Glycemic index: low
Glycemic load: 9
Calories: 76
Protein: 1 gram
Carbohydrates: 18 grams
Fiber: 2 grams
Fat: 0 grams
Saturated fat: 0 grams

2 TB. honey

2 TB. fresh mint, chopped

2 tsp. grated lime peel

2 nectarines, halved, pitted, and cut into ½-inch slices

2 peaches, halved, pitted, and cut into ½-inch slices

½ cantaloupe or other melon, seeded, peeled, and cut into ½-inch cubes

1 cup seedless grapes

Juice of 1 lime

1. In a small bowl, stir together honey, mint, and lime peel. Set aside.

2. In a serving bowl, combine nectarines, peaches, and melon. Cut grapes in half and add to bowl. Drizzle fruit with lime juice and stir gently to coat. Drizzle honey mixture on fruit and serve.

Blueberries with Mango

A colorful summer dessert flavored with brandy and honey.

1 TB. brandy

1 TB. fresh lime juice

1 TB. honey

2 large mangoes, peeled and cut into ¾-inch pieces

1 pint blueberries

1. In a medium bowl, combine brandy, lime juice, and honey.

2. Add mangoes and blueberries. Toss to coat.

Yields 4 cups fruit
Prep time: 15 minutes
Cook time: none
Serving size: ²/₃ cup fruit
Each serving:
Glycemic index: low
Glycemic load: 9
Calories: 88
Protein: 1 gram
Carbohydrates: 21 grams
Fiber: 2 grams
Fat: 0 grams
Saturated fat: 0 grams

Tarragon Fruit Cocktail

Oranges, kiwis, pineapple, and strawberries flavored with fresh tarragon.

2 oranges, peeled, segments cut out and diced

2 kiwis, peeled and diced

¾ cup pineapple, diced

¾ cup fresh strawberries, sliced

1 TB. fresh mint, chopped

2 TB. fresh tarragon, chopped

2 TB. sugar

½ tsp. grated lime peel

In a large bowl, mix oranges, kiwi, pineapple, strawberries, mint, sugar, and lime peel.

Variation: If strawberries are out of season, replace with frozen thawed berries: strawberries, raspberries, blackberries.

Yields 6 cups cocktail
Prep time: 15 minutes
Cook time: none
Serving size: 1 cup cocktail
Each serving:
Glycemic index: low
Glycemic load: 10
Calories: 80
Protein: 1 gram
Carbohydrates: 19 grams
Fiber: 2 grams
Fat: 0 grams
Saturated fat: 0 grams

Tasty Tidbits

Fresh tarragon imparts a light, peppery, slightly anise taste, and is very refreshing in salads and with fruit.

Autumn Fruit Compote

Yields 8 cups compote
Prep time: 20 minutes
Cook time: 20 minutes
Serving size: 1 cup fruit, plus 2 TB. liquid
Each serving:
Glycemic index: low
Glycemic load: 25
Calories: 248
Protein: 3 grams
Carbohydrates: 50 grams
Fiber: 7 grams
Fat: 4 grams
Saturated fat: <1 gram

Apples simmered with oranges and mixed dried fruit, given a spicy accent by cinnamon and walnuts.

1 orange	1 cup dried figs
1 lemon	½ cup walnut halves
4 Jonagold apples, peeled, cored, and cut into 16 wedges	¼ cup honey
	1 tsp. ground cinnamon
1 (8-oz,) pkg. mixed dried fruit	3 cups water

1. With vegetable peeler, remove peel in 1-inch-wide strips from orange and lemon. Squeeze 2 tablespoons juice from lemon. Place in a large saucepan.

2. In a saucepan, add apples, dried fruit, figs, walnuts, honey, cinnamon, and water. Over high heat, bring to boiling. Reduce heat, cover, and simmer, stirring occasionally, until apples are tender—about 10–15 minutes.

3. Serve warm or chilled.

Variation: Substitute Granny Smiths, Pink Lady, Fuji, or Gala apples for the Jonagolds.

Home-Cooked Goodness

Serve this compote as a dessert with hearty main dishes. You'll appreciate its satisfying wintery spices and taste.

Chapter 23

Cakes, Cookies, Pies, and More

In This Chapter

- ◆ Satisfying your sweet tooth
- ◆ No artificial sweeteners
- ◆ Eating more healthful desserts

If you love desserts and have an ambitious sweet tooth to satisfy, you'll find this chapter to be especially comforting. Yes, you can enjoy naturally sweet foods and still eat low or medium glycemic!

But a warning: as with all recipes in our cookbook, read the glycemic load for each recipe and eat the recommended serving size to enjoy the health and weight-management benefits of eating based on the glycemic index.

Hazelnut Sponge Cake

An elegant light dessert cake dessert flavored with hazelnuts and vanilla.

8 eggs, separated	1 tsp. vanilla
¼ tsp. salt	10 oz. hazelnuts (filberts)
½ cup sugar	

1. Preheat the oven to 325°F.

2. Butter and flour a 10×15½× 1-inch pan. Process hazelnuts in a food processor or blender until they become a fine powder.

3. In a large bowl, beat egg whites with salt until stiff. In a separate bowl, beat egg yolks until pale yellow and fluffy. Gradually beat sugar and vanilla into egg yolks. Fold mixture into egg whites. Fold in hazelnuts.

4. Pour batter into the pan. Bake 15–20 minutes, or until cake is lightly browned. Remove from the oven and roll with a clean kitchen towel.

5. When cooled, unroll cake, remove the towel and spread inside of roll with your choice of spread or frosting such as unsweetened fruit preserves, light cream cheese, "Lemon, Orange, and Apricot Cream Cheese Spread" from Chapter 9, or others. Roll again and cut in slices.

Variation: Substitute almonds, walnuts, pecans, or macadamia nuts for the hazelnuts.

Yields 1 (10-inch) rolled cake

Prep time: 20 minutes

Cook time: 15–20 minutes

Serving size: 1 (1-inch) slice

Each serving:

Glycemic index: low

Glycemic load: 11

Calories: 321

Protein: 10 grams

Carbohydrates: 23 grams

Fiber: 3 grams

Fat: 21 grams

Saturated fat: 2.5 grams

Home-Cooked Goodness

To roll sponge cake, dust a kitchen towel with a small amount of confectioner's (powdered) sugar. Invert warm sponge cake on towel. Starting at narrow end of cake, roll both towel and cake together. When cake is cool, unroll and spread with filling. Roll again and it's ready to serve.

Strawberry Jelly Roll

A light and fluffy rolled cake sweetened with strawberry preserves.

5 large eggs, separated

½ cup sugar

1 tsp. vanilla

½ cup almond flour

⅔ cup unsweetened strawberry preserves

Yields 1 (10-inch) roll
Prep time: 20 minutes
Cook time: 15–20 minutes
Serving size: 1 (1-inch) slice
Each serving:
Glycemic index: low
Glycemic load: 15
Calories: 175
Protein: 5 grams
Carbohydrates: 29 grams
Fiber: <1 gram
Fat: 4.3 grams
Saturated fat: 1 grams

1. Preheat the oven to 350°F.

2. Line a 10×15½×1-inch baking pan with parchment paper.

3. In a large bowl, with the mixer at high speed, beat egg whites until soft peaks form. Gradually sprinkle in ¼ cup sugar and beat until egg whites are stiff and glossy.

4. In a small bowl, with the mixer at high speed, beat egg yolks with ¼ cup sugar and vanilla until thick—about 8 minutes. Fold in almond flour.

5. Gently fold egg yolk mixture into egg whites. Spoon batter into the pan. Bake 10–15 minutes, or until light brown.

6. Invert cake on a clean kitchen towel sprinkled with confectioner's sugar. Remove the parchment paper. Roll cake in the towel. Let cool. Unroll, spread with preserves. Roll up again and slice to serve.

Home-Cooked Goodness

Purchase almond flour or nut flour make your own. To make 1 cup, process ¾ cup whole almonds in a food processor fitted with a chopping blade. Stop when almonds turn into flour, but before they turn into almond butter.

Almond Crust with Lemon Cream

Yields 1 (9-inch) pie
Prep time: 20 minutes, plus 3 hour chill time
Cook time: 20 minutes
Serving size: 1 slice pie, 1³/₄ inches wide at crust edge
Each serving:
Glycemic index: low
Glycemic load: 1.5
Calories: 126
Protein: 3.5 grams
Carbohydrates: 9 grams
Fiber: 3 grams
Fat: 8.5 grams
Saturated fat: 4.5 grams

Creamy lemon flavor fills the unique almond crust.

1½ cup almonds

1 egg white

¾ cup xylitol

4 egg yolks

5 TB. fresh lemon juice

1½ TB. fresh lemon peel, grated

2 cups whipping cream

2 TB. sugar

1. Preheat the oven to 375°F.

2. Using a food processor fitted with a chopping blade, process nuts until finely chopped, stopping before nuts turn into flour.

3. Beat egg white until stiff. Gradually fold in ¹/₄ cup xylitol. Fold in chopped almonds. Press mixture firmly over bottom and sides of an oiled 9-inch pie pan. Bake crust until lightly browned—about 8–10 minutes. Remove to a rack and cool.

4. Prepare lemon filling: beat egg yolks until light, add ¹/₂ cup xylitol, lemon juice, and lemon peel. Place egg mixture in the top of a double boiler. Fill bottom of the boiler with water. Bring to a low boil over medium-high heat, stirring. Cook until thick.

5. Whip cream with a mixer until stiff, adding sugar gradually.

6. Place a ¹/₂-inch layer whipped cream on baked almond shell. Spread on egg mixture. Top with remaining whipped cream. Refrigerate at least 3 hours, or overnight.

Variation: For lower fat, sustitute frozen nonfat nondairy whipped topping for the whipping cream and omit sugar. Results: 90 calories, 8 grams fat, <1 gram saturated fat.

Glycemic Notes

There isn't a suitable farm-sourced low-fat alternative for whipping cream, so we suggest substituting Cool Whip Free or frozen nonfat nondairy whipped topping. Use it to reduce the amounts of both fat and saturated fat in desserts. The "free" versions don't contain trans fats.

Pineapple Coconut Cream Pie with Brazil Nut Crust

Pineapple and coconut cream pie, accented with toasted Brazil nuts.

¾ cup Brazil nuts

2 TB. sugar

¾ cup xylitol

⅓ cup Hi-Maize Resistant Starch

1 (14-oz.) can coconut milk

1 (20-oz.) can unsweetened crushed pineapple in its own juice, well drained (reserve liquid)

5 egg yolks

2 TB. butter

1 cup flaked coconut

1 cup whipping cream

2 TB. xylitol

Yields 1 (9-inch) pie		
Prep time: 20 minutes		
Cook time: 25 minutes		
Serving size: 1 slice pie, 1³/₄ inches wide at crust edge		
Each serving:		
Glycemic index: low		
Glycemic load: 15		
Calories: 288		
Protein: 3.5 grams		
Carbohydrates: 22.5 grams		
Fiber: 1.5 grams		
Fat: 20.5 grams		
Saturated fat: 12.5 grams		

1. Preheat the oven to 400°F.

2. Using a food processor fitted with a chopping blade, finely chop Brazil nuts. Blend ground nuts with sugar. Using back of a tablespoon or fingers, press mixture against bottom and sides of a 9-inch pie plate.

3. Bake crust until lightly browned—about 8 minutes. Cool.

4. Prepare filling: Mix xylitol and Hi-Maize in a large saucepan. Place coconut milk in 4-cup measuring container. Add enough reserved pineapple juice to equal 2¹/₂ cups. With a wire whisk, stir liquid into xylitol mixture, and bring to boil over medium heat for 1 minute, stirring occasionally to prevent scorching. Remove from heat.

5. Whisk yolks in a mixing bowl. Gradually stir into hot mixture. Stir over low heat for 2 minutes. Remove from heat.

6. Stir in butter. Stir in crushed pineapple and coconut. Pour into crust. Cover surface with plastic wrap and refrigerate at least 3 hours.

7. Before serving, in a mixing bowl, beat whipping cream until soft peaks form. Sprinkle xylitol on cream and whip until stiff peaks form. Spread over pie.

Cappuccino No-Crust Cheesecake

Coffee and cream add flavor to this rich cheesecake.

Yields 12 servings cheesecake
Prep time: 20 minutes
Bake time: 1 hour 15 minutes, plus 3 hours cool time in oven
Serving size: $^1/_{12}$ pie
Each serving:
Glycemic index: low
Glycemic load: 4
Calories: 216
Protein: 10 grams
Carbohydrates: 25 grams
Fiber: <1 gram
Fat: 8.5 grams
Saturated fat: 5 grams

3 TB. instant coffee granules

1 TB. vanilla

1 lb. nonfat cottage cheese

1 lb. nonfat cream cheese

1¼ cups xylitol

1 TB. dark molasses

2 eggs

4 egg whites

6 TB. Hi-Maize Resistant Starch

½ cup melted butter, cooled

2 cups nonfat sour cream

1. Preheat the oven to 325°F.

2. In a small bowl, stir coffee granules with vanilla until coffee dissolves.

3. Place cottage cheese into a mixer bowl. Add cream cheese and beat with an electric mixer until well blended and creamy.

4. Beat in xylitol, molasses, eggs, and egg whites. Beat in Hi-Maize and coffee mixture. Stir in butter and sour cream at low speed.

5. Pour into a lightly greased 9-inch springform pan and bake 1 hour 15 minutes, or until set. Turn oven heat off and let cake cool in oven 3 hours. Chill well before serving.

 Tasty Tidbits

Dark molasses enhances the flavor of the coffee and provides a rich sugary taste.

Carrot Cake with Pecans and Coconut

An unfrosted moist snack cake flavored with cinnamon and pine-apple.

1½ cups stone-ground whole-wheat flour

½ cup Hi-Maize Resistant Starch

2 tsp. cinnamon

2 tsp. baking soda

½ tsp. salt

3 eggs

¾ cup butter

½ cup skim milk

¾ cup xylitol

2 tsp. vanilla

1 cup unsweetened crushed pineapple, well drained

2 cups carrots, grated

½ cup flaked coconut

½ cup pecans, chopped

Yields 1 (9x15-inch) snack cake
Prep time: 20 minutes
Cook time: 45–55 minutes
Serving size: 1 (3×3-inch) square
Each serving:
Glycemic index: low
Glycemic load: 10
Calories: 253
Protein: 5 grams
Carbohydrates: 28 grams
Fiber: 4 grams
Fat: 13.5 grams
Saturated fat: 7 grams

1. Preheat the oven to 350°F.

2. In a mixing bowl, sift together flour, Hi-Maize, cinnamon, baking soda, and salt; set aside.

3. In a mixer, beat eggs. Add butter, skim milk, xylitol, and vanilla. Mix well. Fold flour mixture into egg mixture. Add pineapple, carrots, coconut, and nuts.

4. Line a 9×13-inch baking dish with parchment paper. Pour in batter and bake at 350°F for 45–55 minutes, or until a toothpick comes out clean when inserted.

The Best Oatmeal Cookies Ever

The soaked raisins provide intense vanilla flavor enhanced with cinnamon and molasses.

3 eggs, well beaten	**1 tsp. salt**
1 cup raisins	**1 tsp. ground cinnamon**
1 tsp. vanilla extract	**2 tsp. baking soda**
1 cup butter	**1½ cups long-cooking oatmeal**
1 TB. dark molasses	
1¾ cups xylitol	**½ cup wheat germ**
1 cup pecan flour	**½ cup pecans, chopped**
½ cup Hi-Maize Resistant Starch	

1. Combine eggs, raisins, and vanilla. Cover and let stand for 1 hour.

2. Preheat the oven to 350°F.

3. In a mixer, cream together butter, molasses, and xylitol. Add pecan flour, Hi-Maize, salt, cinnamon, and soda. Mix well. Blend in egg-raisin mixture, oatmeal, wheat germ, and chopped pecans. Dough will be stiff.

4. Drop by heaping teaspoons onto an ungreased cookie sheet. Bake for 10–12 minutes, or until lightly browned.

Yields 6 dozen cookies

Prep time: 20 minutes

Cook time: 10–12 minutes per batch

Serving size: 1 cookie

Each serving:

Glycemic index: low

Glycemic load: 5

Calories: 75

Protein: 1 gram

Carbohydrates: 8 grams

Fiber: 1 gram

Fat: 5 grams

Saturated fat: 2 grams

Tasty Tidbits

These cookies are a crowd pleaser and provide a high-quality, high-fiber, low-glycemic treat.

Shortbread with Pine Nuts

Shortbread flavored with butter and pine nuts.

1 cup whole-wheat flour	**¼ tsp. salt**
1 cup Hi-Maize Resistant Starch	**1 cup butter at room temperature**
1 cup almond flour	**1 cup pine nuts**
1 cup confectioner's sugar	

1. Preheat the oven to 250°F.

2. Sift flour, Hi-Maize, almond flour, confectioner's sugar, and salt together. Add butter and mix well.

3. Flatten dough to about 1-inch thickness in a circle or oblong shape. Put dough on a baking sheet. Mark for cutting into cookies, cutting only halfway through dough. Press pine nuts into top of dough.

4. Bake on the top shelf of oven for 30 minutes, turning the baking sheet after 20 minutes for even cooking.

5. Cool cookies and cut into indicated shapes. Surface will be pale.

Yields 2 dozen cookies
Prep time: 15 minutes
Cook time: 30 minutes per batch
Serving size: 1 cookie
Each serving:
Glycemic index: low
Glycemic load: 6.5
Calories: 244
Protein: 3 grams
Carbohydrates: 13 grams
Fiber: 6 grams
Fat: 20 grams
Saturated fat: 6.5 grams

 Tasty Tidbits

You can add ¼ tsp. red pepper flakes or cayenne to the batter to add a spicy Southwestern flavor to the pine nut shortbread.

Molasses Ginger Cookies

Spice cookies flavored with zingy ginger and rich molasses.

Yields about 4 dozen cookies
Prep time: 30 minutes, plus 3 hours chill time
Cook time: 9 minutes per batch
Serving size: 2 cookies
Each serving:
Glycemic index: low
Glycemic load: 3
Calories: 100
Protein: 1 gram
Carbohydrates: 15 grams
Fiber: 1 gram
Fat: 4 grams
Saturated fat: 3 grams

1¼ cups stone-ground whole-wheat flour

1 cup Hi-Maize Resistant Starch

1½ tsp. baking soda

1 tsp. ground ginger

½ tsp. ground cinnamon

½ cup butter, softened

¾ cup xylitol

¼ cup dark molasses

1 egg

1. In a medium bowl, stir together flour, Hi-Maize, baking soda, ginger, and cinnamon.

2. In a large mixing bowl, cream butter and xylitol with an electric mixer on low speed for 30 seconds. Beat in molasses and egg until combined. Beat in as much flour mixture as you can with a mixer. Stir in any remaining flour mixture. Cover and refrigerate 3 hours, or until easy to handle.

3. Preheat the oven to 350°F. Shape dough into 1-inch balls. Place balls on a parchment-lined cookie sheet or on an ungreased cookie sheet.

4. Bake for 9–11 minutes, or until edges are firm and tops are puffed; do not overbake. Cool on cookie sheet for 1 minute. Transfer to wire racks. Cool.

Home-Cooked Goodness

Spice cookies are favorites at the Holiday season. Purchase stone-ground whole-wheat flour at the health food store if your grocer doesn't stock it.

Flan

Creamy flan flavored with cinnamon tops caramelized sugar sauce.

1½ cups sugar

8 eggs, lightly beaten

4 cups milk

1 stick cinnamon

1 tsp. vanilla

1. Preheat the oven to 300°F.

2. Place ½ cup sugar in a heavy skillet over medium heat. Melt and cook, stirring, until sugar is caramel-colored. Pour into a buttered, shallow, 2-quart casserole dish so mixture covers bottom. Cool.

3. In a large mixing bowl, gradually beat 1 cup sugar into eggs.

4. In a small saucepan, place milk and cinnamon stick. Heat milk to just under boiling. Remove cinnamon. Slowly add hot milk to egg mixture, stirring constantly to not cook eggs. Add vanilla. Slowly pour over caramel in a casserole dish.

5. Place the casserole dish in a baking pan of boiling water and bake 1 hour, or until set. Cool and chill.

Yields 7–8 cups flan
Prep time: 15 minutes
Bake time: 1 hour
Serving size: ½ cup flan
Each serving:
Glycemic index: medium
Glycemic load: 5.5
Calories: 94
Protein: 5 grams
Carbohydrates: 9.5 grams
Fiber: 0 grams
Fat: 4 grams
Saturated fat: 1.5 grams

Glycemic Notes

When adding a hot mixture to beaten eggs, be careful or you could cook the eggs too soon and end up with lumps. Add just a small amount at first, stirring rapidly, and continue to slowly pour in the hot mixture.

Freezer Lemon Cream

A sweet, frozen cream dessert flavored with lemon and almonds.

Yields 4 cups cream
Prep time: 15 minutes, plus freeze time
Cook time: 10 minutes
Serving size: $^1/_2$ cup cream
Each serving:
Glycemic index: low
Glycemic load: 16
Calories: 253
Protein: 4.5 grams
Carbohydrates: 28.5 grams
Fiber: <1 gram
Fat: 13.46 grams
Saturated fat: 7.8 grams

3 eggs, separated

½ cup sugar

½ cup xylitol

Grated rind and juice of 1 lemon

1 TB. sugar

1 cup heavy cream, whipped

½ cup slivered almonds

1. Combine egg yolks, $^1/_2$ cup sugar, xylitol, lemon rind, and lemon juice in top of a double boiler. Heat over hot water, stirring until mixture thickens. Do not boil. Cool.

2. Beat egg whites until frothy. Add 1 tablespoon sugar and beat until stiff. Fold into cooled custard. Fold in whipped cream.

3. Pour into a buttered freezer tray. Sprinkle with almonds and freeze.

Variation: For lower fat, use frozen nonfat nondairy frozen topping in place of heavy cream. Results: 56 calories, 2.2 grams fat, <1 gram saturated fat.

Tiramisu

Creamy cheese and cream mingle with the dark, rich flavors of coffee and chocolate shavings.

1 cup hot espresso or
strongly brewed coffee

1 TB. brandy

1 TB. sugar

18 crisp ladyfingers (5-oz.
total)

½ cup mascarpone cheese

1½ cup part skim milk ricotta
cheese

¼ cup xylitol

1 TB. cocoa powder

Yields 1 (8x8-inch) pan tiramisu	
Prep time: 20 minutes	
Cook time: none	
Serving size: 1 (2.5×2.5-inch) square	
Each serving:	
Glycemic index: medium	
Glycemic load: 20	
Calories: 141	
Protein: 6 grams	
Carbohydrates: 15 grams	
Fiber: 1 gram	
Fat: 6 grams	
Saturated fat: 3.3 grams	

1. In a small bowl, stir coffee, brandy, and sugar until sugar is dissolved. Cool to room temperature. Dip both sides of 9 ladyfingers in coffee mixture. Arrange in a single layer in an 8×8-inch square baking dish.

2. In large mixing bowl, mix mascarpone cheese, ricotta cheese, and xylitol until smooth.. Spread ½ mixture over ladyfingers.

3. Dip 9 remaining ladyfingers into coffee mixture and arrange on top baking dish. Spread with remaining mascarpone mixture. Sprinkle with cocoa powder. Refrigerate at least 3 hours, or overnight.

Tasty Tidbits _____

You can vary the intensity of the coffee flavor by the strength of the brew you add. To intensify the flavor, pulverize a small amount of instant espresso and sprinkle on the layers of ladyfingers.

Baked Rice Pudding

Yields 5 cups pudding
Prep time: 15 minutes
Cook time: 2¹/₂ hours
Serving size: ¹/₂ cup
Each serving:
Glycemic index: low
Glycemic load: 7
Calories: 105
Protein: 3 grams
Carbohydrates: 13 grams
Fiber: <1 gram
Fat: 4.6 grams
Saturated fat: 2.88 grams

This creamy dessert pudding is flavored with lemon and nutmeg and served with raspberries.

¼ **cup basmati rice**	**Small strip of lemon rind**
2 TB. light brown sugar	¹/₈ **tsp. ground nutmeg**
4 TB. butter	¹/₂ **cup raspberries, fresh or frozen**
3¾ cups skim milk	

1. Preheat the oven to 300°F.

2. Butter a 5-cup shallow baking dish. Put rice, sugar, and butter into the baking dish. Stir in skim milk and lemon rind. Sprinkle with nutmeg.

3. Bake for about 2¹/₂ hours, stirring after 30 minutes, and another couple of times during the next 2 hours, until rice is tender and pudding has a thick and creamy consistency.

4. Serve hot, garnished with raspberries (if frozen, thaw before serving).

Home-Cooked Goodness

The pudding lovers in your family will rave about this dessert. To vary the taste, substitute ¼ teaspoon cardamom for the nutmeg.

Sweet Potato Pudding

Cinnamon and cloves bring out the sweetness of the potatoes in this pudding.

1–2 large sweet potatoes (about 1½ lbs.)

3 eggs, lightly beaten

1 cup milk

⅓ cup sugar

¼ cup yellow cornmeal

2 TB. dark molasses

2 TB. butter, melted

1 TB. vanilla

½ tsp. ground cinnamon

⅛ tsp. ground cloves

¼ tsp. salt

½ cup flaked coconut

¾ cup pecans, chopped

Yields 9 cups pudding
Prep time: 25 minutes
Cook time: 1½ hours, plus 30 minutes cool time
Serving size: ½ cup pudding
Each serving:
Glycemic index: low
Glycemic load: 8
Calories: 138
Protein: 2.5 grams
Carbohydrates: 17 grams
Fiber: 2 grams
Fat: 6.5 grams
Saturated fat: 2.22 grams

1. Preheat the oven to 300°F. Lightly grease bottom and sides of a 2-quart square baking dish. Set aside.

2. Peel and coarsely shred sweet potatoes (about 4 cups). In a large bowl, combine eggs, milk, sugar, cornmeal, molasses, butter, vanilla, cinnamon, cloves, and salt. Stir in shredded sweet potato, ½ cup coconut, and ½ cup pecans. Transfer mixture to the prepared baking dish.

3. Bake, uncovered, for 1 hour. Sprinkle with remaining coconut and pecans. Bake, uncovered, for 30 minutes more, or until a knife inserted near center comes out clean. Cool on a wire rack about 30 minutes. Serve warm.

 Tasty Tidbits

Sweet potatoes are truly a versatile low-glycemic starch. This pudding can light up your holiday dinners with its warming tastes.

Cranberry Apple Crisp

Yields 6 cups crisp
Prep time: 20 minutes
Cook time: 50–55 minutes
Serving size: ½ cup crisp
Each serving:
Glycemic index: low
Glycemic load: 15
Calories: 229
Protein: 3 grams
Carbohydrates: 37 grams
Fiber: 3 grams
Fat: 6 grams
Saturated fat: 3.65 grams

Apples and tart cranberries are accented with cinnamon and topped with a crumbly cookie-like mixture.

3 large Granny Smith Apples

3 large Crispin or Jonagold apples

1 TB. dark molasses

½ cup flour

¾ cup dried cranberries

½ cup xylitol

¼ cup Hi-Maize Resistant Starch

½ tsp. cinnamon

6 TB. butter, cut into ½-inch pieces

½ cup apple juice

1. Preheat the oven to 350°F.

2. Peel, core, and slice apples. Place in a large bowl. Add molasses, 1 tablespoon flour, and cranberries. Toss to mix. Pour into a 2-quart baking dish. Pour juice on top.

3. Put xylitol, remaining flour, Hi-Maize, and cinnamon into a food processor fitted with a chopping blade. Pulse a few times to blend. Add butter and pulse until mixture is crumbly. Sprinkle on apple mixture.

4. Bake 50–55 minutes until top is browned and apples are tender. Serve warm or at room temperature.

Home-Cooked Goodness

Fragrant apple pie is everyone's favorite. The cranberries give it a tangy surprise. Serve by itself or with a slice of cheddar cheese, a spoonful of heavy cream, or a dollop of vanilla ice cream.

Chapter 24

Chocolate Desserts

In This Chapter

- Lower-glycemic chocolate desserts
- Using quality chocolate
- Savoring the entire experience

If you love chocolate, most likely you've been stumped about how to eat your chocolate and eat low glycemic, too. With these recipes, you'll discover many wonderful, delicious, and quite frankly decadent ways to do just that.

Our recipes include cakes, cookies, mousses, and flavored ganache for toppings and fillings. Not all of the recipes are low glycemic, but they're lower glycemic than their high-glycemic counterparts.

Chocolate-Lovers' Ingredients

We're picky about our chocolate, and most likely you are, too. Here's a list of quality ingredients to use in these recipes in order to get the best flavor from your chocolate desserts:

- Unsweetened cocoa powder. We like Hershey's. It's widely available and has a rich taste.

- Xylitol is a healthful sugar alcohol that bakes and tastes like sugar.

- Dark molasses gives a rich sugar taste with fewer calories than brown sugar. You don't need much.

- Butter. Use real dairy butter. Margarines and vegetable oils can't deliver the flavor and excellence you want.

- Dairy products—full fat, low-fat, or nonfat. It's your choice based on your desired fat intake. Both work in most recipes unless the recipe directions call for whipping the cream. The only nonfat viable alternative to whipped cream we've found is Cool Whip Free, which is a frozen nonfat nondairy whipped topping.

- Ten-pound chocolate bars. If you're really into chocolate, find a baking supply store that sells 10-pound bars. Some brand names you can purchase are Guittard, Callebaut, Ghiradelli, and Merckins. Bars come in several varieties of white, milk, semisweet, and bittersweet. A bar can last months and the price per pound is lower than purchasing bags of chocolate chips.

- Parchment paper is a baker's best friend. No more oiling and flouring pans. Line your baking pans with it. It pulls free with no sticking.

- Hi-Maize is a high-*amylose* corn flour that works well as a partial substitute for flour. It has a lower glycemic value and contains good-for-your-gut fiber.

def•i•ni•tion

Amylose is a type of dietary starch found in plants that is lower in glycemic value than amylopectin, the other type of plant-based starch.

- Oat bran is high in fiber, nutritious, and added to some of our cookie recipes to give you an added health bonus.

- Eggs. Use whole eggs. If the recipe calls for whole eggs or egg yolks, don't skimp and use only egg whites—the dessert won't deliver full flavor and satisfaction.

 Glycemic Notes

Pay close attention to the recommended serving size for our chocolate desserts. They aren't large, so eat slowly. Savor each bite. Favor your waistline and not your appetite.

With these high-quality ingredients, you're on your way to having your chocolate and eating it, too.

Chocolate Sponge Cake

A light vanilla flavor accents the rich chocolate taste of this cake.

4 eggs

1 cup xylitol

1½ TB. butter, melted

¼ cup unsweetened cocoa powder

1 tsp. vanilla

4 TB. water

1 tsp. flour

⅓ cup Hi-Maize Resistant Starch

1 TB. unsweetened cocoa powder

Yields 1 (9-inch) cake
Prep time: 20 minutes
Cook time: 50 minutes
Serving size: 1 wedge slice, 2⅓ inches wide at edge
Each serving:
Glycemic index: low
Glycemic load: 1
Calories: 67
Protein: 3 grams
Carbohydrates: 7 grams
Fiber: 1 gram
Fat: 3 grams
Saturated fat: 1 gram

1. Preheat the oven to 350°F.

2. Lightly grease a 9-inch cake pan and line base with waxed paper or parchment paper.

3. In an electric mixer, beat eggs until fluffy, then gradually add xylitol and beat for 15 minutes.

4. Combine butter, cocoa powder, vanilla, and water. Fold into egg mixture. Sprinkle flour over egg mixture. Add Hi-Maize and gently fold into eggs. Spoon mixture into the prepared cake pan.

5. Bake for approximately 50 minutes or until just firm to the touch. When cooled, dust with 1 tablespoon cocoa powder.

Tasty Tidbits _____

Serve this light chocolate cake with coffee or tea and fresh fruit for dessert.

Flourless Chocolate Layer Cake

Raspberries accent the dark chocolate layer cake.

Yields 1 (9-inch) torte	
Prep time: 25 minutes	
Cook time: 30–35 minutes	
Serving size: 1 wedge slice, 1 inch wide at edge	
Each serving:	
Glycemic index: 38 low	
Glycemic load: 6	
Calories: 193	
Protein: 3 grams	
Carbohydrates: 16 grams	
Fiber: <1 gram	
Fat: 13 grams	
Saturated fat: 7.3 grams	

8 oz. bittersweet chocolate, chopped	6 egg yolks
1 cup butter, softened	8 egg whites
½ cup sugar	4 TB. unsweetened raspberry jam or jelly
½ cup xylitol	1 TB. powdered sugar
2 TB. flour	1 cup fresh raspberries

1. Preheat the oven to 350°F.

2. Fit 2 (9-inch) round cake pans with parchment paper. In a small saucepan over low heat, cook and stir bittersweet chocolate until melted. Let cool for 10 minutes.

3. In a large bowl, beat butter with an electric mixer on medium to high speed for 30 seconds. Add sugar, xylitol, and flour. Beat until combined. Beat in melted chocolate. Add egg yolks, 2 at a time, beating well after each addition.

4. Thoroughly wash the beaters, rinse in cool water, and dry. In another large bowl, beat egg whites with an electric mixer on medium speed until peaks are stiff.

5. Stir some egg white into chocolate mixture. Gently fold rest of egg whites into chocolate mixture. Divide batter evenly between the pans.

6. Bake for 30–35 minutes, or until tops spring back when lightly touched and a toothpick inserted near centers comes out clean. Cool in the pans on a wire rack for 10 minutes. Remove cake from the pans; cool completely.

7. To serve, spread jam on top of one cake layer. Top with second cake layer. Sprinkle with powdered sugar. Garnish with fresh raspberries.

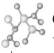

Glycemic Notes

This layer cake is high in fat. Be sure to enjoy every bite and budget it into your daily fat intake allowance.

Chocolate Zucchini Pound Cake

A moist pound cake flavored with orange, cinnamon, chocolate, and walnuts.

¾ cup butter

1½ cups xylitol

3 eggs

2 tsp. vanilla

2 tsp. orange peel, grated

2 cups zucchini, peeled and coarsely shredded

1 cup flour

1 cup oat bran

1 cup walnut flour

2½ tsp. baking powder

1½ tsp. baking soda

1 tsp. salt

1 tsp. cinnamon

½ cup skim milk

2 (1-oz.) squares unsweetened baking chocolate, grated

Yields 1 (10-inch) tube pan
Prep time: 20 minutes
Cook time: 1 hour
Serving size: 1 wedge-shaped slice, 1¾ inch at edge
Each serving:
Glycemic index: low
Glycemic load: 7
Calories: 208
Protein: 2 grams
Carbohydrates: 23 grams
Fiber: 1 gram
Fat: 11 grams
Saturated fat: 5.7 grams

1. Preheat the oven to 350°F. Oil and lightly flour a 10-inch tube pan.

2. With an electric mixer, beat together butter and xylitol. Add eggs one at a time, beating well after each addition.

3. With a large spoon, stir in vanilla, orange peel, and zucchini.

4. In a mixing bowl, stir together flour, oat bran, walnut flour, baking powder, soda, salt, and cinnamon. Add flour mixture to batter, alternating with milk. Stir in grated chocolate.

5. Pour into the tube pan and bake for 1 hour.

Tasty Tidbits

Zucchini and walnut flour keep this cake moist, rich, and flavorful.

Chocolate Date Nut Snack Cake

Chocolate is baked into and sprinkled on this moist cake.

Yields 16 squares
Prep time: 15 minutes
Cook time: 40–50 minutes
Serving size: 1 (2.75×2.75-inch) square
Each serving:
Glycemic index: low
Glycemic load: 6
Calories: 191
Protein: 2 grams
Carbohydrates: 21 grams
Fiber: 3 grams
Fat: 11 grams
Saturated fat: 3.45 grams

¾ cup hot water

½ cup dates, cut into quarters

¾ cup almonds

½ cup (1 stick) butter

½ cup xylitol

2 eggs

½ cup Hi-Maize Resistant Starch

1 tsp. baking soda

2 TB. cocoa powder

1 tsp. vanilla extract

½ cup semisweet chocolate morsels

½ cup walnuts

1. Preheat the oven to 350°F. Line a 9×9-inch baking pan with parchment paper.

2. In a small mixing bowl, add hot water to dates and let cool.

3. Process ¾ cup almonds in a food processor to make 1 cup almond flour. In a mixer, cream butter with xylitol. Add eggs and beat until smooth.

4. Mix in almond flour, Hi-Maize, baking soda, cocoa, and vanilla. Stir in date mixture. Blend thoroughly.

5. Pour batter into the prepared pan. Sprinkle with chocolate chips and nuts. Bake for 40–50 minutes or until top springs back when lightly pressed with your finger.

Tasty Tidbits _____

Dates add moisture and sweetness to this rich and satisfying chocolate cake.

Chocolate Chip Cookies

Chocolate morsels and vanilla flavor this all-time favorite cookie.

½ cup whole wheat flour

½ cup oat bran

½ tsp. salt

½ tsp. baking soda

1 cup Hi-Maize Resistant Starch

¾ cup (1½ sticks) butter at room temperature

2 TB. dark molasses

½ cup xylitol

2 eggs

1½ tsp. vanilla extract

1 cup semisweet chocolate morsels

Yields 4 dozen cookies
Prep time: 20 minutes
Cook time: 8–10 minutes per batch
Serving size: 1 cookie
Each serving:
Glycemic index: low
Glycemic load: 3
Calories: 45
Protein: 1 gram
Carbohydrates: 7 grams
Fiber: 1 gram
Fat: 1.5 grams
Saturated fat: .75 grams

1. Preheat the oven to 375°F.

2. In a side bowl, mix together flour, oat bran, salt, baking soda, and Hi-Maize.

3. Cream butter, dark molasses, and xylitol in a large bowl with an electric mixer. Add eggs and vanilla and blend. Add dry ingredient blend to butter mixture and mix until uniform. Add chocolate morsels and mix.

4. Drop by teaspoonfuls onto an ungreased cookie sheet.

5. Bake 8–10 minutes.

Variation: Add 1 cup chopped walnuts when you add the chocolate morsels.

 Home-Cooked Goodness _____

Everyone loves chocolate chip cookies. These will please your family and be more healthful, too.

Flourless Cherry Chip Cookies

Yields 4 dozen cookies
Prep time: 25 minutes
Cook time: 9 minutes per batch
Serving size: 1 cookie
Each serving:
Glycemic index: low
Glycemic load: 6
Calories: 114
Protein: 1 gram
Carbohydrates: 15 grams
Fiber: 1.5 grams
Fat: 5.5 grams
Saturated fat: 3 grams

Home-Cooked Goodness

Oatmeal adds to the crunchy quality of these cookies.

Chocolate chips and cherries flavor crunchy drop cookies.

1 cup butter, softened
½ cup sugar
3 TB. dark molasses
½ cup xylitol
1 tsp. baking soda
1 tsp. salt
2 eggs

1½ tsp. vanilla
1 cup pecan flour
1 cup oatmeal
1 cup Hi-Maize Resistant Starch
1 (12-oz.) pkg. semisweet chocolate pieces
1 cup dried cherries

1. Preheat the oven to 375°F.

2. In a large mixing bowl, beat butter with sugar, molasses, xylitol, baking soda, and salt. Beat until combined.

3. Beat in eggs and vanilla until combined. Slowly beat in pecan flour, oatmeal, and Hi-Maize. Batter will be thick. Stir in chocolate morsels and cherries.

4. Drop dough by tablespoons 2 inches apart onto an ungreased cookie sheets. Bake 8–10 minutes until slightly browned. Transfer cookies to racks.

Cream Cheese Marbled Brownies

Sweet chocolate and tangy cream cheese are whirled together with vanilla and almond flavors.

Yields 16 brownies
Prep time: 25 minutes
Cook time: 40–50 minutes
Serving size: 1 (2.25×2.25-inch) brownie
Each serving:
Glycemic index: low
Glycemic load: 6
Calories: 196
Protein: 2 grams
Carbohydrates: 20 grams
Fiber: 1 gram
Fat: 12 grams
Saturated fat: 5 grams

1 (4-oz.) bar German chocolate

5 TB. butter

1 (3-oz.) pkg. cream cheese

1 cup xylitol

3 eggs

1 TB. and ¼ cup Hi-Maize Resistant Starch

1 tsp. vanilla extract

¼ cup flour

½ tsp. baking powder

½ tsp. salt

½ cup walnuts, chopped

1 tsp. vanilla extract

¼ tsp. almond extract

1. Preheat the oven to 350°F. Line a 9×9-inch baking pan with parchment paper.

2. Melt chocolate and 3 tablespoons butter in the top of double boiler. Set aside to cool.

3. In a medium-size bowl, cream 2 tablespoons butter and cream cheese until fluffy. Blend ¼ cup xylitol, 1 egg, 1 tablespoon Hi-Maize, and 1 teaspoon vanilla into creamed mixture and set aside.

4. In another bowl, beat 2 eggs and add ¾ cup xylitol. Sift ¼ cup Hi-Maize, flour, baking powder, and salt into eggs. Stir melted chocolate, walnuts, vanilla, and almond extract into egg mixture.

5. Spread ½ chocolate mixture evenly in bottom of a greased 9×9-inch pan. Spread cream cheese mixture over chocolate layer. Drop spoonfuls of remaining chocolate over cream cheese layer. Swirl with a fork for marbled effect.

6. Bake for 40–50 minutes, or until a toothpick comes out clean.

Tasty Tidbits

German chocolate has been processed to remove the natural acidity of the chocolate so that it's alkaline. This gives the chocolate a deeper color, but a softer taste.

Lucy's Brownies

Dark, rich, chocolatey brownies flavored with vanilla or your choice of variation.

Yields 30 brownies
Prep time: 20 minutes
Cook time: 20–30 minutes
Serving size: 1 brownie, about 2×2 inches
Each serving:
Glycemic index: low
Glycemic load: 5
Calories: 116
Protein: 3 grams
Carbohydrates: 15 grams
Fiber: 1 gram
Fat: 9 grams
Saturated fat: 4.9 grams

1½ sticks butter

1 cup xylitol

¼ cup sugar

2 TB. dark molasses

4 eggs

1 tsp. vanilla

½ tsp. salt

1 cup pecan flour

2 TB. Hi-Maize Resistant Starch

1 cup Hershey's unsweetened cocoa powder

½ cup chocolate morsels

1. Preheat the oven to 350°F. Line a 9×13-inch baking dish with parchment paper.

2. In an electric mixer, cream butter, xylitol, sugar, and molasses. Add eggs 1 at a time, beating well after each addition until batter is smooth. Add vanilla and mix well.

3. Add salt, pecan flour, Hi-Maize, and cocoa powder. (Add additional seasoning variation, if desired, here.) Mix until smooth. Stir in chocolate chips.

4. Turn batter into the pan. Bake for 20–30 minutes. Cool on rack. Invert and remove the parchment paper. Return to the pan.

Variations: Hot and spicy: Add ½ to 1 teaspoon cayenne or hot chili powder.
Spicy: Add ½ to 1 teaspoon freshly ground black pepper.
Mocha: Add ½ to 1 teaspoon instant coffee powder.
Fruit: Add ½ cup raisins, dried cranberries, or dried cherries.
Coconut: Add ½ cup shredded coconut.
Tarragon: Add ½ to 1 teaspoon dried tarragon.
Ginger: Add 2–3 tablespoons chopped candied ginger.
Morsels: Substitute butterscotch, white chocolate, cherry-flavored, or mint chocolate morsels.

Tasty Tidbits

From Lucy: Every one of these variations is superb. My favorite is black pepper with or without instant coffee. My friends prefer the pecan flour to wheat flour, because the brownies are moister and richer.

Chocolate Fluff Parfait

Bittersweet chocolate blended with whipped cream and flavored with vanilla.

3 oz. bittersweet chocolate

4 egg yolks

1¼ tsp. vanilla extract

4 egg whites, room temperature

4 cups whipped cream

Yields 7 cups parfait
Prep time: 20 minutes
Cook time: 4 minutes
Serving size: ¹/₃ cup
Each serving:
Glycemic index: low
Glycemic load: 2
Calories: 179
Protein: 1.5 grams
Carbohydrates: 5 grams
Fiber: <1 gram
Fat: 17 grams
Saturated fat: 11.8 grams

1. In the top of a double boiler over simmering water, melt chocolate. Cool. Add egg yolks, 1 at a time, mixing well after each. Beat with whisk until light. Stir in ¹/₄ teaspoon vanilla. Cool.

2. In an electric mixer, beat egg whites until soft peaks form. Gradually add powdered sugar and ¹/₂ teaspoon vanilla. Continue beating until stiff peaks form. Fold melted chocolate mixture into egg whites. Volume will decrease. Set aside in a cool place.

3. Fold ¹/₂ whipped cream into chocolate mixture. Spoon layer of whipped cream into bottom of champagne-style stemmed glasses, reserving ¹/₄ cup for decoration. Divide chocolate mixture evenly among the glasses. Spoon remaining cream on top. Refrigerate until ready to serve.

Variation: For lower fat, substitute frozen nonfat nondairy whipped topping for the whipped cream. Results: 44 calories, 2 grams fat, 1 gram saturated fat.

Home-Cooked Goodness

Bar chocolate tastes different than chocolate morsels (and we think better), because forming a morsel that will hold its shape during shipping and stocking requires a different formulation. To achieve the purest chocolate taste, use bittersweet bar chocolate for this recipe.

Chocolate Ganache

Rich, creamy, sensuous chocolate sauce for toppings and fillings.

Yields 1½ cups ganache	
Prep time: 5 minutes	
Cook time: 2 minutes	
Serving size: 1 TB.	
Each serving:	
Glycemic index: low	
Glycemic load: 1	
Calories: 56	
Protein: <1 gram	
Carbohydrates: 3.5 grams	
Fiber: <1 gram	
Fat: 4.6 grams	
Saturated fat: 2.91 grams	

6 oz. (about 1 cup) bitter-sweet (about 70%) chocolate   **½ cup heavy cream**

1. Coarsely chop chocolate; set aside.

2. In a medium saucepan, scald cream over medium-high heat. Remove from heat immediately.

3. Add chocolate (do not stir). Let stand 5 minutes. Stir until smooth. Cool 10 minutes.

4. Serve as a topping for ice cream and custards. Add a dollop on cake or brownies. Use as a filling or frosting for cakes. To serve as fudge or candy, refrigerate in a square 9×9-inch pan, cut into squares, and serve.

Variations: Add one of the following to accent the flavor of the chocolate:

¼ tsp. dried tarragon

¼ tsp. fresh chopped basil

⅛ tsp. freshly ground black pepper

⅛ tsp. red pepper flakes

⅛ tsp. grated lemon, lime, or orange peel

1 TB. dried or fresh cherries, chopped

1 TB. fresh pineapple, chopped

⅛ tsp. dried coriander

⅛ tsp. ground ginger, or 1 TB. fresh chopped candied ginger

1 tsp. fresh mint, chopped, or ¼ tsp. peppermint or spearmint extract

1 TB. brandy or liqueur such as Amaretto, Kirsch, Kahlua, Schnapps

1 tsp. instant coffee crystals (add to cream while scalding)

1 tsp. Earl Grey tea leaves, finely chopped

1 TB. grated chocolate nibs

Glycemic Notes

Be sure to eat ganache sparingly and lovingly. A little goes a long way. While it's low glycemic, it does contain plenty of calories and saturated fat.

Pots de Crème

An elegant and easy-to-make chocolate mousse with rum flavoring.

1 cup 2 percent milk, heated to boiling point

1 cup semisweet or bitter-sweet chocolate morsels

1 large egg

2 TB. sugar

2 TB. rum or favorite liqueur

Fresh fruit, whipped cream, chocolate curls, or unsweetened cocoa powder

1. Combine milk, chocolate, egg, sugar, and rum in a food processor or blender. Blend on high until chocolate is melted and smooth. Pour into 6 pots de crème or demitasse cups. Chill until firm.

2. Garnish with a piece of fruit, dollop of whipped cream, chocolate shavings, or cocoa powder, if desired.

Yields 2 cups mousse
Prep time: 10 minutes
Cook time: 2–3 minutes
Serving size: 1/3 cup mousse
Each serving:
Glycemic index: low
Glycemic load: 11
Calories: 206
Protein: 3 grams
Carbohydrates: 26 grams
Fiber: 1 gram
Fat: 10 grams
Saturated fat: 6 grams

Tasty Tidbits

No one will know how quick and easy this is to prepare, and the taste is mouthwatering and decadent.

White Chocolate Mousse

Creamy, cold white chocolate flavored with vanilla and a hint of lemon.

Yields 6 cups mousse
Prep time: 15 minutes
Cook time: 5 minutes
Serving size: 1/4 cup mousse
Each serving:
Glycemic index: low
Glycemic load: 3
Calories: 109
Protein: 1.5 grams
Carbohydrates: 10 grams
Fiber: <1 gram
Fat: 7 grams
Saturated fat: 4 grams

12 oz. Guittard's white chocolate, chopped (Do not use coating chocolate. Guittard's is made with cocoa butter.)

3/4 cup milk

1 TB. unflavored gelatin

1/4 cup milk, warmed

2 1/2 tsp. vanilla extract

4 large egg whites, room temperature

1/8 tsp. salt

2 cups heavy cream, whipped

1/8 tsp. fresh lemon juice

1. Melt white chocolate in 3/4 cup milk in top of a double boiler over hot, not boiling, water. (White chocolate melts at a low temperature and will become "grainy" if heated too much.) Stir until smooth and remove from heat.

2. Soften gelatin in 1/4 cup warmed milk, stirring until dissolved. Add gelatin to chocolate, stirring constantly until smooth. Stir in vanilla. Cool to room temperature.

3. In a small bowl, beat egg whites until foamy. Add salt and continue beating until stiff peaks form. Mix 1/3 whites into chocolate mixture. Gently fold in remaining whites in 2 additions.

4. Fold whipped cream into chocolate mixture in 3 additions. Stir in lemon juice. Pour into a glass serving bowl. Chill at least 3 hours before serving.

Variation: For lower fat, use 2 percent milk and replace whipped cream with frozen nonfat nondairy whipped topping. Results: 96 calories, 5.6 grams fat, 3.2 grams saturated fat.

Home-Cooked Goodness

A wonderful dessert made without sugar or flour. Serve with grated chocolate, fresh berries, or mint sprigs.

Chocolate-Walnut Mousse

Creamy milk chocolate mousse flavored with cognac and topped with bittersweet chocolate.

1 (6-oz.) pkg. milk chocolate morsels

½ cup skim milk

2 tsp. unflavored gelatin

2 TB. cold water

2 eggs, separated

⅛ tsp. salt

⅛ tsp. cream of tartar

2 TB. sugar

¼ cup cognac

1 cup heavy cream, whipped

½ cup toasted walnuts, chopped

2 TB. bittersweet chocolate morsels, melted and cooled

½ tsp. instant coffee powder

Walnut halves

Yields 5 cups mousse
Prep time: 25 minutes, plus chill overnight
Cook time: 5 minutes
Serving size: ¼ cup mousse
Each serving:
Glycemic index: low
Glycemic load: 3
Calories: 112
Protein: 1.5 grams
Carbohydrates: 8.5 grams
Fiber: <1 gram
Fat: 8 grams
Saturated fat: 4.2 grams

1. Day before: Combine chocolate and milk in a heavy saucepan and heat over very low heat, stirring occasionally, until chocolate melts.

2. Soften gelatin in water.

3. Beat egg yolks lightly and add a little hot chocolate mixture. Return mixture to the saucepan and cook, stirring, until chocolate-egg mixture thickens slightly. Do not boil. Stir softened gelatin into hot chocolate mixture until dissolved. Cool to room temperature.

4. With an electric mixer, beat egg whites with salt and cream of tartar until stiff. Gradually beat in sugar.

5. Stir cognac into cooled chocolate mixture. Fold in egg whites, 1 cup whipped cream, and walnuts. Turn into a serving bowl. Cover and chill overnight.

6. Next day: Fold melted square of chocolate and coffee powder into remaining whipped cream. Spoon on top of chilled mousse. Decorate with walnut halves.

Chocolate Mousse with Raspberry Sauce

Yields 4 cups plus ³/₄ cup raspberry sauce
Prep time: 20 minutes, plus 1 hour chill time
Cook time: 2–3 minutes
Serving size: ¹/₄ cup mousse plus 1¹/₂ TB. raspberry sauce
Each serving:
Glycemic index: low
Glycemic load: 7
Calories: 132
Protein: 1 gram
Carbohydrates: 17 grams
Fiber: <1 gram
Fat: 6.7 grams
Saturated fat: 6.3 grams

Intense raspberry flavor highlights a deep chocolate mousse.

¾ cup unsweetened raspberry jam

1 TB. raspberry liqueur or unsweetened fruit juice

3 oz. semisweet chocolate

1 oz. (1 square) bitter baking chocolate

2 TB. honey

1 TB. brandy or unsweetened fruit juice

2½ cups Cool Whip

Chocolate curls or grated chocolate

1. In a small saucepan, heat jam over low heat until melted, stirring occasionally. Remove from heat. Stir in raspberry liqueur or juice and set aside to cool completely.

2. In another small saucepan, heat chocolate over low heat until melted and smooth. Remove from heat. Stir in honey, and brandy or juice., until well combined. Transfer mixture to a large bowl and set aside to cool completely.

3. Fold Cool Whip into chocolate mixture.

4. Spoon chocolate mixture into 6 wine glasses or dessert dishes. Spoon cooled raspberry sauce over mousse and top with chocolate curls. Cover and chill for 1–6 hours.

Variation: For lower fat, use Cool Whip Free frozen nonfat nondairy whipped topping for whipping cream. Results: 72 calories, <1 gram fat, <1 gram saturated fat.

Home-Cooked Goodness

Choose from many flavors of unsweetened juice—raspberry, cranberry, pomegranate, blueberry, and cherry—as a replacement for the liqueur in this recipe.

Chocolate Cinnamon Chiffon Pie

A Brazil-nut crust filled with fluffy cinnamon-flavored chocolate.

1 envelope unflavored gelatin	**1 tsp. vanilla extract**
¼ cup xylitol	**2 TB. sugar**
¼ tsp. salt	**1 tsp. cinnamon**
1 cup milk	**½ cup heavy cream, whipped**
2 eggs, separated	**Brazil Nut Crust (see Chapter 23 "Desserts")**
1 cup (6-oz. pkg.) semisweet chocolate pieces	

1. Combine gelatin, xylitol, and salt in top of a double boiler. Stir in milk, egg yolks, and chocolate pieces. Place over boiling water and cook, stirring constantly, until gelatin has dissolved and chocolate is melted—about 6 minutes.

2. Remove from heat and water. Beat with a rotary beater until chocolate is blended. Stir in vanilla and chill about 1 hour.

3. With an electric mixer, beat egg whites in a small bowl until stiff but not dry. Gradually add sugar and cinnamon and beat until stiff. Fold into gelatin mixture. Fold in whipped cream.

4. Turn mixture into Brazil-nut crust and chill until firm. Garnish with additional whipped cream and sprinkle with chopped Brazil nuts.

Yields 1 (9-inch) pie
Prep time: 20 minutes, plus 1 hour chill time
Cook time: 6 minutes
Serving size: 1 pie wedge, 1¾ inches wide at back edge

Each serving:
Glycemic index: low
Glycemic load: 4
Calories: 136
Protein: 1.5 grams
Carbohydrates: 13.5 grams
Fiber: <1 gram
Fat: 5.25 grams
Saturated fat: 3 grams

Tasty Tidbits

South of the border, cinnamon is often blended with chocolate in beverages and sauces. Cinnamon can be helpful in reducing high blood sugar levels.

Chocolate No-Crust Cheesecake

A rich, deep cheesecake that will thoroughly satisfy any chocolate lover.

Yields 24 servings cheesecake	

Prep time: 20 minutes

Bake time: 1 hour 15 minutes, plus 3 hours cool time in oven

Serving size: 1 slice 1 inch wide at back

Each serving:

Glycemic index: low

Glycemic load: 3

Calories: 227

Protein: 5 grams

Carbohydrates: 18 grams

Fiber: 1 gram

Fat: 15.4 grams

Saturated fat: 7.5 grams

1 lb. cottage cheese

1 lb. cream cheese

1¼ cups xylitol

4 eggs

1 cup part skim milk ricotta cheese

12 oz. bittersweet or semi-sweet chocolate, broken into small pieces and melted

1 TB. cocoa powder

1 tsp. vanilla extract

1 cup sour cream

1. Preheat the oven to 325°F.

2. Place cottage cheese into a mixer bowl. Add cream cheese and beat with an electric mixer until well blended and creamy.

3. Beat in xylitol, and eggs. Beat in ricotta cheese until smooth. Stir in melted chocolate, cocoa powder, vanilla extract, and sour cream at low speed.

4. Pour into a lightly greased 9-inch springform pan and bake 1 hour 15 minutes, or until set. Turn the oven heat off and let cake cool in the oven 3 hours. Chill well before serving.

Home-Cooked Goodness

Lower the fat content in this recipe by using low-fat cottage cheese or cream cheese, but not both. If you use both, you'll lose the creamy mouth feel and satisfying taste of the cheesecake.

Resources

Most of the ingredients in our recipes can be purchased at a grocery store. If not, look for them at a health food store. In addition, if you want more information on the glycemic index, we provide some helpful resources here.

Where to Purchase Specialty Items

Some ingredients are specialty items. Here's a list of where to purchase them:

◆ Coarse cornmeal is sold in the health food section of grocery stores or natural food stores or purchased online.

◆ Steel-cut oats for oatmeal is available at health food stores and specialty food markets.

◆ Chocolate bars. Most large cities have baker supply stores that stock a good selection of 10-pound bars. You can also purchase online at grchocolates.stores.yahoo.net/larchocbar.html. Order chocolate to be sent to you only during the winter months; otherwise it could melt in shipment.

◆ Hi-Maize Resistant Starch can be ordered at www.amazon.com and at www.kingarthurflour.com. It comes in 5-pound bags.

◆ Kashi cereal is sold at grocery stores.

◆ Oat bran is sold in the health food section of grocery stores or natural food stores or purchased online.

◆ Stevia Plus is widely available at grocery stores and health food stores. You can also purchase at www.amazon.com.

◆ Stone-ground whole-wheat flour is sold in the health food section of grocery stores or natural food stores or purchased online.

◆ Rye flour is sold in the health food section of grocery stores or natural food stores.

◆ Xylitol is sold in the health food section of grocery stores or natural food stores and can be purchased online.

Information on the Glycemic Index

To learn more about the glycemic index. Use these resources:

◆ **www.glycemicindex.com.** This website is from the originators of the glycemic index at the University of Sydney in Australia.

◆ **www.glycemicindex.com.** You can subscribe to GI News, which is an e-mail newsletter.

◆ **www.mendosa.com.** A site for people with diabetes to learn how to manage blood sugar with the glycemic index.

Index

F

NEWLY REVISED by Lucy Beale and Joan Clark-Warner, M.S., R.D., C.D.E.

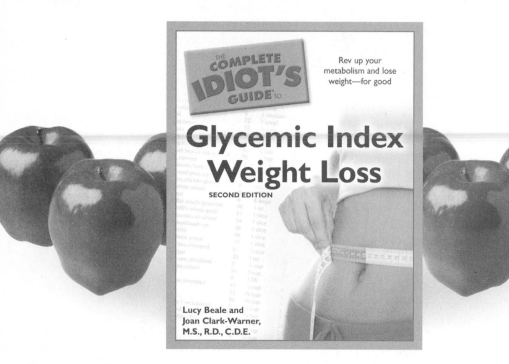

The Complete Idiot's Guide® to Glycemic Index Weight Loss, Second Edition, provides a solid foundation for understanding just how and why a glycemic index diet works and controlling counts along with activity and stress levels. In this fully updated and expanded edition, you will learn everything you need to know about:

- The basics of body chemistry, metabolism, and insulin.
- Planning and starting a weight loss program including setting goals, counting carbs, balanced eating, exercise, snacking, shopping, eating out, and more.
- Information on supplements, basic easy recipes, food lists, and sample meal plans.
- A full appendix with glycemic index counts and loads for all sorts of foods.
- The new study on eating certain foods cold—and why that makes a big difference.

ALPHA   idiotsguides.com